KT-570-952

OXFORD MEDICAL PUBLICATIONS

Liver and Pancreatobiliary Surgery

with Liver Transplantation

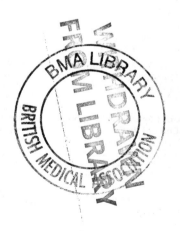

Oxford Specialists Handbooks published and forthcoming

General Oxford Specialist Handbooks
A Resuscitation Room Guide
Addiction Medicine
Hypertension
Perioperative Medicine, Second Edition
Post-Operative Complications, Second edition

Oxford Specialist Handbooks in Anaesthesia
Cardiac Anaesthesia
General Thoracic Anaesthesia
Neuroanaesthesia
Obstetric Anaesthesia
Paediatric Anaesthesia
Regional Anaesthesia, Stimulation and Ultrasound Techniques

Oxford Specialist Handbooks in Cardiology
Adult Congenital Heart Disease
Cardiac Catheterization and Coronary Intervention
Echocardiography
Fetal Cardiology
Heart Failure
Hypertension
Nuclear Cardiology
Pacemakers and ICDs

Oxford Specialist Handbooks in Critical Care
Advanced Respiratory Critical Care

Oxford Specialist Handbooks in End of Life Care
End of Life Care in Cardiology
End of Life Care in Dementia
End of Life Care in Nephrology
End of Life Care in Respiratory Disease
End of Life in the Intensive Care Unit

Oxford Specialist Handbooks in Neurology
Epilepsy
Parkinson's Disease and Other Movement Disorders
Stroke Medicine

Oxford Specialist Handbooks in Paediatrics
Paediatric Endocrinology and Diabetes
Paediatric Dermatology
Paediatric Gastroenterology, Hepatology, and Nutrition
Paediatric Haematology and Oncology
Paediatric Nephrology
Paediatric Neurology
Paediatric Radiology
Paediatric Respiratory Medicine

Oxford Specialist Handbooks in Psychiatry
Child and Adolescent Psychiatry
Old Age Psychiatry

Oxford Specialist Handbooks in Radiology
Interventional Radiology
Musculoskeletal Imaging

Oxford Specialist Handbooks in Surgery
Cardiothoracic Surgery
Hand Surgery
Oral Maxillofacial Surgery
Operative Surgery, Second Edition
Otolaryngology and Head and Neck Surgery
Plastic and Reconstructive Surgery
Surgical Oncology
Urological Surgery
Vascular Surgery

✍ www.oup.co.uk/academic/medicine/osh/

Oxford Specialist Handbooks in Surgery

Liver and Pancreatobiliary Surgery

with Liver Transplantation

Robert P. Sutcliffe
Specialist Registrar,
General Surgery,
South East Thames Deanery, UK

Charalambos Gustav Antoniades
Specialist Registrar in Hepatology,
Institute of Liver Studies,
King's College Hospital,
London, UK

Rahul Deshpande
Specialist Registrar in Hepatobiliary Surgery,
Institute of Liver Studies,
King's College Hospital, UK

Olga N. Tucker
Senior Lecturer in Surgery,
University of Birmingham,
Birmingham, UK

Nigel Heaton (Senior Author)
Consultant Surgeon,
Liver Transplant Surgical Service,
King's College Hospital,
London, UK

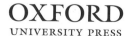

OXFORD
UNIVERSITY PRESS

OXFORD
UNIVERSITY PRESS

Great Clarendon Street, Oxford OX2 6DP

Oxford University Press is a department of the University of Oxford.
It furthers the University's objective of excellence in research, scholarship,
and education by publishing worldwide in

Oxford New York

Auckland Cape Town Dar es Salaam Hong Kong Karachi
Kuala Lumpur Madrid Melbourne Mexico City Nairobi
New Delhi Shanghai Taipei Toronto

With offices in

Argentina Austria Brazil Chile Czech Republic France Greece
Guatemala Hungary Italy Japan Poland Portugal Singapore
South Korea Switzerland Thailand Turkey Ukraine Vietnam

Oxford is a registered trade mark of Oxford University Press
in the UK and in certain other countries

Published in the United States
by Oxford University Press Inc., New York

British Library Cataloguing in Publication Data
Data available

Library of Congress Cataloging-in-Publication-Data
Liver and pancreatobiliary surgery with liver transplantation/Robert Sutcliffe . . .
[et al.]; Nigel Heaton (senior author).
     p. ; cm. — (Oxford specialist handbooks in surgery)
ISBN 978–0–19–920538–7 (alk. paper)
1. Liver—Surgery—Handbooks, manuals, etc. 2. Pancreas—Surgery—Handbooks,
manuals, etc. 3. Biliary tract—Surgery—Handbooks, manuals, etc. I. Sutcliffe, Robert,
Dr. II Heaton, Nigel, III. Series: Oxford specialist handbooks in surgery.
     [DNLM: 1. Liver Diseases—Surgery—Handbooks. 2. Biliary Tract Diseases—Surgery—
Handbooks. 3. Liver Transplantation—methods—Handbooks.
4. Pancreatic Diseases—Surgery—Handbooks. WI 39 L7834 2009]
     RD546. L5545 2009
     617.5'562059—dc22   2009019007

Typeset by Cepha Imaging Private Ltd., Bangalore, India
Printed in China
on acid-free paper through
Asia Pacific Offset
ISBN 978–0–19–920538–7

10 9 8 7 6 5 4 3 2 1

Preface

Hepatobiliary and pancreatic surgery has grown significantly as a surgical speciality over the last 20 years. The realization that patients with colorectal liver metastases can be cured by surgery has led to a marked increase in the number of liver resections performed worldwide. We have seen improved short-term outcomes due to advances in both surgical techniques and perioperative care, while the advent of effective adjuvant chemotherapeutic agents and locoregional therapies, such as radiofrequency ablation, have contributed to excellent long-term results.

Attention has turned to the management of hepatocellular carcinoma, which usually arises on a background of cirrhosis. The indications for liver resection and transplantation for this condition are continually being refined, and in selected patients with localized disease and favourable tumour biology, five-year survival rates of more than 70% have been consistently achieved. Locoregional and systemic therapies including biological agents are proving valuable adjuncts in both the adjuvant and palliative settings.

Progress in the management of cholangiocarcinoma and pancreatic cancer is the next major challenge that lies ahead for clinicians who are involved in the care of patients with hepatobiliary disease. Major liver and pancreatic resections can now be performed with low mortality and acceptable morbidity in high volume specialist centres. Aggressive surgical management can provide long-term survival for selected patients with cholangiocarcinoma, a disease that was previously considered to have a dismal prognosis. For patients with more advanced disease, their outlook will remain poor unless effective systemic treatments become available.

For surgeons in training, hepatobiliary and pancreatic surgery remains an exciting and dynamic specialty that demands a high level of surgical expertise, and a thorough knowledge and understanding of anatomical and pathological principles. The key to successful patient outcomes is through multimodal therapies orchestrated by a cohesive multidisciplinary team approach. Pursuit of a career in this field is a great challenge, but equally rewarding, and I hope that this handbook will provide a comprehensive insight into the diagnosis and management of hepatobiliary and pancreatic surgical diseases in an accessible format.

Contents

Detailed contents

Symbols

📖	cross references
↑	increased
↓	decreased
→	leading to
❶	warning
▶	important

Abbreviations

AAA	abdominal aortic aneurysm
AIH	autoimmune hepatitis
ALD	alcohol-related liver disease
ALF	acute liver failure
ALP	alkaline phosphatase
ALT	alanine aminotransferase
AMA	antimitochondrial antibody
ANA	antinuclear antibody
AP	acute pancreatitis
AR	acute rejection
ARDS	acute respiratory distress syndrome
ASA	American Society of Anesthesiologists
ASIS	anterior superior iliac spine
ASMA	anti-smooth muscle antibody
AST	aspartate aminotransferase
BCLC	Barcelona Clinic Liver Cancer
BCS	Budd-Chiari syndrome
bd	twice daily
BD	bile duct
BDI	bile duct injury
BP	blood pressure
CA	cystic artery
CAH	chronic active hepatitis
CASH	chemotherapy-associated steatohepatitis
CASR	calcium-sensing receptor
CBD	common bile duct
CCK	cholecystokinin
CD	cystic duct
CHA	common hepatic artery
CHD	common hepatic duct
CLIP	Cancer of the Liver Italian Program
CLM	colorectal liver metastases
CMV	cytomegalovirus
CO	carbon monoxide
COPD	chronic obstructive pulmonary disease
CP	chronic pancreatitis

CPP	cerebral perfusion pressure
CPR	cardiopulmonary resuscitation
CPS	cardiopulmonary support
CT	computed tomography
CUSA	Cavitron ultrasonic aspirator
CVP	central venous pressure
EBV	Epstein-Barr virus
ECG	echocardiogram
ECMO	extracorporeal membrane oxygenation
EHBA	extrahepatic biliary atresia
ELAD	extracorporeal liver assist devices
EN	enteral nutrition
ER	emergency room
ERCP	endoscopic retrograde cholangiopancreatography
ES	endoscopic sphincterotomy
EUS	endoscopic ultrasound
FBC	full blood count
FDG	2-fluoro-2-deoxy-D-glucose
FFP	fresh frozen plasma
FL	falciform ligament
FLR	future liver remnant
FNH	focal nodular hyperplasia
G&S	group and save
GB	gallbladder
GCS	Glasgow Coma Score
GGT	gamma glutamyl transpeptidase
HAS	human albumin solution
HAT	hepatic artery thrombosis
HBV	hepatitic B virus
HCC	hepatocellular carcinoma
HDU	high dependency unit
HDV	hepatitis delta virus
HIDA	hepatobiliary iminodiacetic acid
HIV	human immunodeficiency virus
HPB	hepato pancreatobiliary
HR	heart rate
HV	hepatic vein
HVEPC	hepatic vascular exclusion with preservation of caval flow
HVPG	hepatic venous pressure gradient
IBD	inflammatory bowel disease

ICP	intracranial pressure monitor
IHIVC	infrahepatic inferior vena cava
IM	intramuscular
INR	international normalized ratio
IOUS	intraoperative ultrasonography
IPMT	intraductal papillary mucinous tumour
ITP	idiopathic thrombocytopaenic purpura
ITU	intensive care unit
IV	intravenous
IVC	inferior vena cava
IVDU	intravenous drug users
JIS	Japan Integrated Staging
JPS	Japanese Pancreatic Society
LDH	lactate dehydrogenase
LFT	liver function tests
LHA	left hepatic artery
LHD	left hepatic duct
LHV	left hepatic vein
LIF	left iliac fossa
LMW	low molecular weight
LPV	left portal vein
LRV	left renal vein
LTL	left triangular ligament
LUS	laparoscopic ultrasonography
MAP	mean arterial pressure
MDMA	methylenedioxymethamphetamine
MELD	Model for End-stage Liver Disease
MHV	middle hepatic vein
MODS	multiple organ dysfunction syndrome
MOF	multi-organ failure
MRCP	magnetic resonance cholangiopancreatography
MRI	magnetic resonance imaging
MRSA	methicillin resistant *Staphylococcus aureus*
NADH	nicotinamide adenine dinucleotide
NAFLD	non-alcoholic fatty liver disease
NASH	non-alcoholic steatohepatitis
NBM	nil by mouth
NCNNE	non-colorectal non-neuroendocrine liver metastases
NET	neuroendocrine tumours
NHBD	non-heart beating donor

NOM	non-operative management
NSAID	non-steroidal anti-inflammatory drug
OCP	oral contraceptive pill
od	once a day
OLT	orthotopic liver transplant
PAC	pulmonary artery catheter
PAF	platelet activating factor
PanIN	pancreatic intraepithelial neoplasia
PBC	primary biliary cirrhosis
PCWP	pulmonary capillary wedge pressure
PD	pancreaticoduodenectomy (Ch 11)
PEI	percutaneous ethanol injection
PET	positron emission tomography
PFIC	progressive familial intrahepatic cholestasis
PGE_2	prostaglandin E2
PiCCO	pulse contour cardiac output
po	per oral (by mouth)
PPPD	pylorus preserving pancreaticoduodenectomy
prn	pro re nata (as required)
PSC	primary sclerosing cholangitis
PTC	percutaneous transhepatic cholangiography
PV	portal vein
PVE	portal vein embolization
qds	four times daily
RFA	radiofrequency thermal ablation
RHA	right hepatic artery
RHD	right hepatic duct
RHV	right hepatic vein
RPV	right portal vein
RRV	right renal vein
RTL	right triangular ligament
RUQ	right upper quandrant
SAAG	serum/ascites albumin gradient
SaO_2	O_2 arterial saturation
SBP	spontaneous bacterial peritonitis
SC	subcutaneous
SFS	small for size syndrome
SHIVC	suprahepatic inferior vena cava
SIRS	systemic inflammatory response syndrome
SjO_2	reverse jugular oxygen saturation

SMA	superior mesenteric artery
SMV	superior mesenteric vein
SOD	sphincter of Oddi
SPEN	solid and papillary epithelial neoplasm
SPPT	solid pseudo-papillary tumour
SRS	somatostatin receptor scintigraphy
TACE	transarterial chemo-embolization
TAP	trypsinogen activation peptide
TAUSS	transabdominal ultrasonography
TB	tuberculosis
TCP	tropical chronic pancreatitis
tds	three times daily
TEG	thromboelastography
TIPS	transjugular intrahepatic portosytemic shunt
TNF	tumour necrosis factor
TNM	tumour node metastasis
TOE	transoesophageal echocardiography
TVI	total vascular isolation
U&E	urea and electrolytes
UC	ulcerative colitis
UCSF	University of California, San Francisco
UDCA	ursodeoxycholic acid
UKELD	UK Model for End-stage Liver Disease
UW	University of Wisconsin solution
VEGF	vascular endothelial growth factor

List of Contributors

Narendra Battula
Specialist Registrar in General Surgery
West Midlands Deanery, UK

Paolo Muiesan
Consultant Liver Transplant Surgeon
Queen Elizabeth Hospital, UK

Natalie Philips
Specialist Registrar in Gastroenterology
Charing Cross Hospital, UK

Tasmeen Pirani
Specialist Registrar in Gastroenterology
London, UK

Anatomy and physiology

R. Sutcliffe & O. Tucker

Liver segmental anatomy

- The liver is the largest solid organ (weight 1.2–1.6kg), and lies in the right upper quadrant of the abdomen below the right hemidiaphragm.
- **Peritoneal attachments:** falciform ligament, coronary ligament, and left and right triangular ligaments (see Fig. 1.3).
- The **Glissonian capsule** is a fibrous covering over the liver, except the *bare area*, where the liver is in direct contact with the diaphragm.

Liver segments

- Anatomical divisions are based on vascular and biliary anatomy not surface markings (see Figs 1.1 and 1.2).
- The arterial supply to the liver is via the **common hepatic artery** (branch of coeliac axis), which usually runs to the left of the common bile duct, before dividing into left and right branches. There is considerable anatomical variation of the hepatic arteries (Hepatic artery anatomy 📖 p. 6).
- The **mid-plane of the liver** separates the **right lobe** (supplied by right hepatic artery and right portal vein) from the **left lobe** (supplied by left hepatic artery and left portal vein). The principal plane (see Fig. 1.1) intersects the gallbladder fossa anteriorly and the inferior vena cava fossa posteriorly.
- The left and right hepatic ducts (**first-order ducts**) drain bile into the common hepatic duct from each lobe.
- **Second-order ducts** and arteries divide each lobe into two *sections.*
  - right lobe => anterior and posterior sections;
  - left lobe => medial and lateral sections.
- The left intersectional plane corresponds to the umbilical fissure and the attachment of the falciform ligament to the liver. The right intersectional plane does not have a surface marking.
- **Third-order divisions** of the liver are also known as Couinaud's segments.
  - right anterior section => segments 5 and 8
  - right posterior section => segments 6 and 7;
  - left lateral section => segments 2 and 3;
  - left medial section => segment 4.
- The **caudate lobe** is distinct from the left and right lobes, and is also referred to as segment 1. It lies between the porta hepatis and the inferior vena cava. It receives a blood supply from both left and right hepatic arteries, and bile drains into both left and right hepatic ducts.

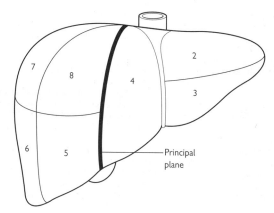

Fig. 1.1 Principal plane.

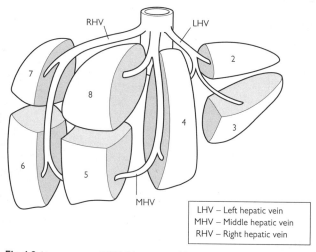

Fig. 1.2 Liver segments. LHV: left hepatic vein, MHV: middle hepatic vein, RHV: right hepatic vein.

- The **portal vein** drains blood from the gastrointestinal tract (from lower oesophagus to rectum), pancreas, and spleen. It is formed by the union of the splenic and superior mesenteric veins posterior to the neck of the pancreas. The inferior mesenteric vein invariably drains into the splenic vein.
- The **right portal vein** supplies the right lobe and its branches correspond to those of the right hepatic artery.
- The **left portal vein** is initially *horizontal* and changes direction at the **ligamentum venosum** to become *vertical* (umbilical portion, in the umbilical fissure). The vertical portion is a remnant of the umbilical vein, and gives branches to segment 4 (to its right), and segments 2 and 3 (to its left).
- The **hepatic veins** drain blood from the liver into the *inferior vena cava*, and lie between sections or lobes:
  - *left hepatic vein* – between s2 and s3 then left intersectional plane;
  - *middle hepatic vein* – mid-plane (between s4 and s5/8);
  - *right hepatic vein* – right intersectional plane (between s5/8 and s6/7).
- 10% of patients have a large inferior right hepatic vein in addition to a superior right hepatic vein.
- The caudate lobe drains blood directly into the IVC, via several small veins.

See Fig. 1.3.

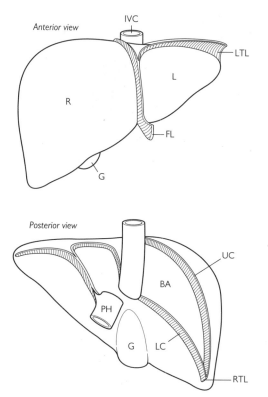

Fig. 1.3 Peritoneal attachments of the liver. G: gallbladder, FL: falciform ligament, LTL: left triangular ligament, IVC: inferior vena cava, R: right lobe, L: left lobe, PH: porta hepatis, BA: bare area, UC: upper layer of coronary ligament, LC: lower layer of coronary ligament, RTL: right triangular ligament.

Hepatic artery anatomy

- An **accessory artery** indicates that the proper hepatic artery (left, right, or common) is also present.
- A **replaced artery** indicates that the proper artery is absent.
- An **accessory** or **replaced left hepatic artery** arises from the left gastric artery and runs in the lesser omentum.
- An **accessory** or **replaced right hepatic artery** arises from the superior mesenteric artery, and passes behind the common bile duct to run along its right posterolateral border into the liver.

Liver resection planes

- **Anatomical liver** resections follow anatomical planes (Fig. 1.4).
- Transection through umbilical fissure/falciform ligament
  (*left intersectional plane*):
  - left lateral sectionectomy (or 'segmentectomy');
  - extended right hepatectomy.
- Transection through *mid-plane*:
  - left hepatectomy;
  - right hepatectomy.
- Transection through *right intersectional plane*:
  - extended left hepatectomy;
  - right posterior sectionectomy.

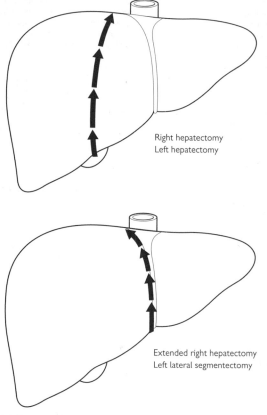

Right hepatectomy
Left hepatectomy

Extended right hepatectomy
Left lateral segmentectomy

Fig. 1.4 Resection planes.

Liver physiology

- The liver parenchyma is arranged into *lobules*, which contain several *acini*. An acinus is arranged around terminal branches of the hepatic artery and portal vein.
- Hepatocytes receive their blood supply via the *hepatic sinusoids*, which are fenestrated capillaries lined by endothelial cells. Sinusoids are lined by *Kupffer cells* (part of reticulo-endothelial system), *hepatic stellate cells*, and liver-associated lymphocytes.
- Bile canaliculi drain bile from hepatocytes into a network of cholangioles and larger ducts, before entering the common hepatic duct

Liver function

The liver has substantial reserve capacity, which allows significant damage (e.g. cirrhosis) to occur before symptoms develop. A significant volume of liver (up to 60%) can be resected safely, without patients developing liver failure, provided that the future liver remnant is of good quality and an adequate volume (see Complications after liver resection, Early, Small-for-size syndrome 📖 p. 190).

- **Metabolism:**
  - carbohydrates (gluconeogenesis, glycogenesis, glycogenolysis);
  - protein;
  - lipids;
  - bilirubin;
  - hormones;
  - haemoglobin;
  - drugs;
  - lactate.
- **Synthesis:**
  - albumin;
  - clotting factors (fibrinogen, prothrombin, V, VII, IX, XI, protein C, protein S, antithrombin);
  - cholesterol;
  - triglycerides;
  - bile;
  - lipoproteins;
  - caeruloplasmin;
  - transferrin;
  - complement;
  - glycoproteins.
- **Storage**
  - glycogen;
  - vitamin B12;
  - iron;
  - copper.
- **Foetal erythropoiesis.**

Gallbladder anatomy

- The gallbladder is a hollow organ that concentrates and stores bile. It lies in the gallbladder fossa on the inferior aspect of the right lobe. It has a rounded *fundus,* a body, and an *infundibulum.* Gallstones may become impacted in *Hartmann's pouch.*
- The presence of fat in the duodenum stimulates the release of *cholecystokinin (CCK),* which causes contraction of the gallbladder and secretion of bile through the cystic duct, common bile duct, and into the duodenum.
- **Calot's triangle** is bordered by the gallbladder, the common hepatic duct and the liver (Fig. 1.5). The peritoneal covering of the gallbladder extends onto the anterior and posterior aspects of Calot's triangle and onto the portal structures. The arterial supply of the gallbladder is via the *cystic artery,* which usually arises from the right hepatic artery and lies within *Calot's triangle.* Occasionally, the cystic artery has anterior and posterior branches before entering the gallbladder.
- The **cystic duct** joins the common hepatic duct to form the common bile duct, usually about 5cm above the duodenum. Rarely, an accessory cystic duct (duct of Luschka) drains bile intrahepatically through the gallbladder fossa, and is susceptible to injury during cholecystectomy (Fig. 1.6).
- Venous drainage of the gallbladder occurs via multiple small veins that enter the portal vein, either through the gallbladder fossa or Calot's triangle

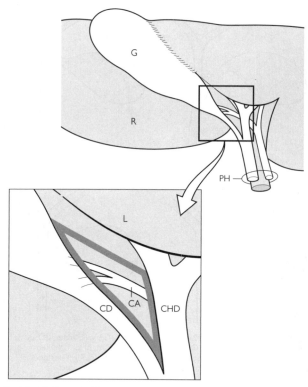

Fig. 1.5 Calot's triangle. PH: porta hepatis, R: right lobe of liver, G: gallbladder, L: liver, CD: cystic duct, CHD: common hepatic duct, CA: cystic artery.

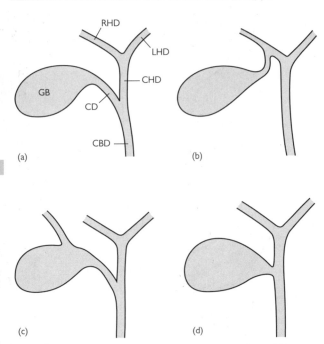

Fig. 1.6 Gallbladder anatomical variation. (a) Normal (GB: gallbladder; CD: cystic duct; CBD: common bile duct; CHD: common hepatic duct; RHD: right hepatic duct; LHD: left hepatic duct). (b) Cystic duct draining into RHD. (c) Right posterior sectoral duct draining into gallbladder. (d) Short or absent cystic duct.

Biliary anatomy

- The left and right hepatic ducts unite at the base of segment 4, anterior to the portal vein bifurcation. The common hepatic duct passes inferiorly in the right edge of the *hepatoduodenal ligament*, to the right of the common hepatic artery, and joins the cystic duct to become the common bile duct.
- The common bile duct (diameter 3–7mm) passes behind the first part of the duodenum, enters the head of the pancreas, and terminates at the ampulla of Vater.
- Many anatomical variants of biliary anatomy have been described (Fig. 1.7).
- The blood supply of the biliary tree is derived principally from the hepatic artery, which explains the presence of biliary complications that develop after hepatic artery thrombosis in liver transplant recipients.

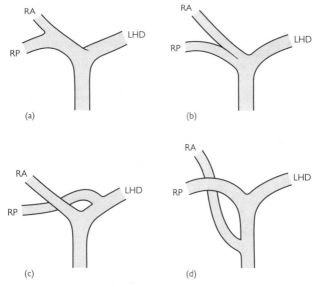

Fig. 1.7 Hepatic duct anatomical variation. (a) Normal anatomy (RA: right anterior sectoral duct, RP: right posterior sectoral duct, LHD: left hepatic duct). (b) Right anterior and posterior sectoral ducts drain directly into confluence (c) Right posterior sectoral duct drains into left hepatic duct. (d) Right anterior sectoral duct drains into common hepatic duct.

Pancreatic anatomy

- The pancreas is a retroperitoneal organ, which is separated from the stomach anteriorly by the lesser sac. It consists of a head, neck, body and tail. The head of the pancreas lies within the C-shaped duodenum. The neck lies at the level of the first lumbar vertebra (transpyloric plane of Addison), anterior to the confluence of the portal, superior mesenteric and splenic veins, and connects to the body and tail. The tail of the pancreas is closely related to the splenic hilum within the *lienorenal ligament*.
- The *uncinate process* of the pancreas originates from the embryological dorsal pancreas and fuses with the pancreatic head (ventral pancreas). It lies posterior to the superior mesenteric artery and vein.
- Exocrine secretions (see Fig.1.8) enter the pancreatic duct (diameter 1-3mm) that joins with the accessory pancreatic duct and the common bile duct to form a common channel that terminates at the ampulla of Vater (postero-medial border of the second part of the duodenum).
- The arterial supply of the pancreas is via branches of the coeliac axis (gastroduodenal artery => superior pancreatico-duodenal artery), superior mesenteric artery (inferior pancreatico-duodenal artery) and branches directly from the splenic artery.
- Venous drainage is via tributaries into the splenic, portal and superior mesenteric veins.
- Lymphatic drainage of the pancreas occurs via lymph nodes located along the arterial supply (coeliac axis and superior mesenteric artery).

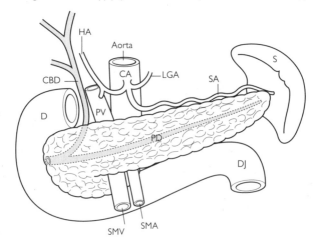

Fig. 1.8 Anatomical relationships of the pancreas. D: duodenum, S: spleen, CBD: common bile duct, PD: pancreatic duct, DJ: duodeno-jejunal flexure, PV: portal vein, SMV: superior mesenteric vein, HA: hepatic artery, SA: splenic artery, SMA: superior mesenteric vein, CA: coeliac axis.

Pancreatic physiology

- **Exocrine:** acinar cells secrete bicarbonate (regulated by secretin) and inactive pro-enzymes (regulated by CCK), which are activated in the duodenum (e.g. trypsin, amylase, lipase, chymotrypsin). Bicarbonate neutralizes gastric acid, and enzymes digest dietary proteins, lipids, and carbohydrate to allow absorption. Lipid absorption is facilitated by bile acids (secreted in bile).
- **Endocrine:** Islets of Langerhans consist of alpha, beta, delta, and PP cells, which secrete *glucagon, insulin, somatostatin*, and *pancreatic polypeptide*, respectively.

Investigation of liver and pancreatobiliary disease

C. Antoniades, N. Philips, T. Pirani, & O. Tucker

General approach

- The choice of imaging modality may be influenced by local availability of expertise and facilities.
- Investigations should be guided by clinical presentation and suspected diagnosis/differential diagnosis. A thorough history and physical examination are therefore essential steps in guiding further investigations and management. Baseline liver function tests and liver ultrasound are mandatory first-line investigations in all patients.

Symptoms and signs

The following scenarios require different diagnostic pathways, and will be covered in subsequent chapters.

Patient with suspected liver disease

- Risk factors for viral hepatitis (blood transfusion, tattoos, IV drug abuse, foreign travel).
- Detailed history of alcohol consumption.
- Drug history.
- Symptoms of chronic liver disease (jaundice, encephalopathy, ascites, oedema).
- Family history of liver disease.
- Peripheral stigmata of chronic liver disease (spider naevi, palmar erythema, leukonychia, clubbing, jaundice).
- Portal hypertension (variceal bleed, ascites, splenomegaly, caput medusae).
- Kayser-Fleischer rings (Wilson's disease).

See Parenchymal liver disease 📖 p. 53.

Patient with liver lesion

- Age and sex.
- Oral contraceptive use (FNH, adenoma).
- Anabolic steroid use (FNH, adenoma).
- Previous treatment for endometriosis (FNH).
- Symptoms/signs of cirrhosis, including Child-Pugh score (hepatocellular carcinoma).
- Symptoms/history of gastrointestinal malignancy.
- Previous malignancy (e.g. breast cancer, melanoma).
- Fever, malaise, foreign travel (abscess).

See Liver lesions 📖 p. 133.

Patient with obstructive jaundice

- Exclude cirrhosis/hepatitis.
- Exclude intrahepatic cholestasis (drugs, sepsis).
- Intermittent (stones) or progressive (malignancy).
- Painful (stones) or painless (malignancy).
- Fevers (cholangitis).
- Weight loss (malignancy).
- Cachexia (advanced malignancy).
- Vomiting (duodenal obstruction due to malignancy).
- Abdominal distension/ascites (peritoneal metastases).

- Previous HPB surgery (e.g. cholecystectomy or biliary bypass).
- Level of duct dilatation on US (e.g. hilar = probable cholangiocarcinoma vs. distal CBD = stones vs. pancreatic tumour).
- Gallstones on US (does not exclude malignancy).

See Bile duct obstruction 📖 p. 208.

Patient with bile leak or iatrogenic bile duct injury after cholecystectomy

- Timing of cholecystectomy.
- Details of initial operation.
- Immediate or delayed recognition.
- Presence of sepsis.
- Adequate drainage of collections.
- Extent/nature of injury (cholangiography).
- Associated arterial injury (CT angiography).

See Laparoscopic cholecystectomy, Complications 📖 p. 227.

Patient with pancreatic lesion

- Age.
- Comorbidity.
- History of previous malignancy, especially renal carcinoma (metastasis).
- Recent onset of diabetes.
- History of multiple endocrine neoplasia (e.g. pituitary, parathyroid tumours, family history).
- Imaging characteristics of lesion (solid vs. cystic, size, relation to pancreatic duct).

See Pancreatic adenocarcinoma 📖 p. 262, Cystic lesions 📖 p. 270.

Baseline tests

Liver function tests

Biochemical tests of liver function are important to determine the cause and extent of underlying disease. They are useful in selecting patients who require a liver biopsy and follow-up.

- **'Hepatic enzymes':**
  - alanine aminotransferase (ALT);
  - aspartate aminotransferase (AST).
- **'Biliary enzymes':**
  - alkaline phosphatase (ALP)
  - gamma glutamyl transpeptidase (GGT)
- **Synthetic function:**
  - International normalised ratio (INR);
  - albumin.
- **Bilirubin transport:** bilirubin (conjugated and unconjugated) and metabolism.

Deranged liver function tests

- **Drugs:** non-steroidal anti-inflammatory drugs, steroids, paracetamol, antibiotics, statins, anti-epileptics, anti-tuberculosis treatment, illicit drugs, herbal preparations.
- **Infection:** viral hepatitis (A/B/C, EBV, CMV),
- **Hereditary:** haemochromatosis.
- **Alcohol.**
- **Obesity:**
  - fatty liver;
  - non-alcoholic steatohepatitis (NASH).
- **Autoimmune:**
  - primary biliary cirrhosis;
  - primary sclerosing cholangitis.
- **Biliary obstruction:**
  - cholangitis;
  - choledocholithiasis;
  - cholangiocarcinoma;
  - gallbladder carcinoma;
  - pancreatic carcinoma;
  - benign biliary stricture;
  - choledochal cyst.

Transaminitis

- Raised ALT and AST suggests viral hepatitis, alcoholic liver disease, non-alcoholic steatohepaitis, autoimmune disease.
- Alcohol: AST/ALT ratio >2, raised MCV, thrombocytopenia, raised GGT.

Cholestasis

- **Raised ALP/GGT:** PBC, PSC, biliary stricture, malignancy (cholangiocarcinoma, carcinoma head of pancreas).
- **Isolated elevation of ALP:** consider bone disease.
- **Isolated elevation of GGT:** common and should be investigated if persistently rising or other LFT abnormalities.

Transabdominal ultrasound

Description

A tomographic imaging technique that provides anatomical + functional imaging with high resolution without the need for contrast agents by placing a transducer probe on the abdominal wall.

The technology of ultrasound scanning

- Ultrasound is a high frequency, mechanical vibration with alternate waves of compression + rarefaction.
- Ultrasound waves are generated by piezo-electric crystals in a transducer which focuses the waves into a beam.
- Commonly used frequencies for non-endoscopic TAUSS range from 3.5 to 5MHz.
- The higher the frequency the better the spatial resolution.
- The majority of the beam is reflected as it crosses tissues of different acoustic properties, termed acoustic impedence determined by tissue density + rigidity.
- The small proportion of the beam that is absorbed by the tissue dissipates as heat.
- The image is created from the reflected sound beam returning to the transducer.
- The delay between sending the pulse + detection of the returning echo, + its direction from the transducer is used to calculate the depth of the reflecting surface.

Echopattern

- **Echofree:** when ultrasound waves pass through fluid no reflection occurs (ascites, fluid collection) + these areas appear black with posterior enhancement.
- **Echogenic:** when ultrasound waves pass through solid structures (e.g. calculi, bone) the majority of the sound waves are reflected + appear as white with posterior shadowing.
- The strength of the echoes is proportional to the change in acoustic impedance at the tissue interface.

Scanner types

- **Real time:** the beam is rapidly swept through the tissue to be examined, repeated 10–30 times/s to give a moving image.
- **Linear array:** the beam is swept along an area 2cm wide × 5–10cm long. This technique displays superficial structures better than real time scanners.
- **Curved linear array:** combines methods used in linear array + real time scanners.

Additional techniques

Doppler
- Colour Doppler: provides a non-invasive image of vascular anatomy.
- Spectral or pulsed Doppler: used to assess velocity of flow providing functional information on blood flow.
- Duplex scanning: simultaneous combination of imaging with Doppler.

Contrast-enhanced transabdominal ultrasonography
- Intravenous injection of microbubbles as ultrasound contrast agents. Microbubbles are confined to the vascular compartment.
- Composed of a gas, air, or perfluoro compound, surrounded by a stabilizing shell, phospholipids, surfactant, or denatured albumin.
- <7µM in diameter to allow them to cross the capillary beds.
- The technique is dependent on the difference in compressibility of the gases within the microbubbles compared with the incompressibility of tissue.
- Can be used to improve Doppler studies, termed Doppler rescue.
- Contrast specific imaging techniques use the principles of Doppler, phase modulation, amplitude modulation, or a combination both modulation approaches.

Ultrasound-guided biopsy
Methods
- Freehand.
- Needle guided.

Advantages
- Rapid investigation.
- Non-invasive.
- Allows real time imaging.
- Low cost.
- Provides structural detail down to 1mm.
- Interactive: signs can be elicited during transabdominal ultrasonography (TAUSS) permitting a targeted approach, e.g. acute cholecystitis, acute appendicitis.
- Imaging can be performed in any plane.
- Well tolerated procedure.
- No preparation required.
- Can be performed at the patients bedside: hand-held devices for use in the emergency room (ER), portable devices for use in the intensive care unit (ICU).
- Can be used to plan or perform procedures, e.g. marking the appropriate site for paracentesis.
- Can be used to perform tissue biopsies under no or local anaesthetic.

Disadvantages
- Operator dependent.
- Cannot be readily reviewed.
- Suboptimal quality in the obese.
- Repetition for follow-up can be difficult if performed by different operators or at wide time intervals.

Indications for transabdominal ultrasonography
Liver
- **Assessment of liver size:** normal – left lobe span 5–10cm, right lobe span 8–15cm.
- **Assessment of diffuse liver disease:**
  - fatty infiltration;

- acute hepatitis;
- cirrhosis.
- **Focal liver lesion:**
  - size;
  - solitary or multiple;
  - segmental distribution;
  - relationship to biliary + vascular structures;
  - echopattern;
  - differential diagnosis determined by characteristics of lesion.
- **Assessment of segmental anatomy** prior to lesional biopsy, resection, or ablation.
- **Assessment of hepatic vasculature:**
  - *portal vein* – portal hypertension with demonstrable collaterals, portal vein thrombosis;
  - *hepatic artery* – hepatic artery thrombosis;
  - *hepatic veins* – Budd Chiari syndrome, veno-occlusive disease, congestive hepatomegaly;
  - intrahepatic vascular shunts;
  - inferior vena cava: patency after conventional liver transplantation, thrombosis, stricture.
- **Assessment of intrahepatic biliary radicals:**
  - *diameter* – dilation, stricture;
  - *content* – stones, parasites.

Extrahepatic biliary tree
- **Gallbladder:**
  - *Size* –
    - *normal* – long axis 6–12cm, short axis 3–5cm;
    - *contracted* – ≤5cm.
    - *distended* – ≥12cm (after prolonged fast).
  - *Wall thickness* – normal: ≤3mm thick.
  - *Content* – calculi, microlithiasis (sludge), parasites, pus (empyema), mucus (mucocoele).
  - *Mural lesion* – polyps, carcinoma.
- **Cystic duct:**
  - diameter;
  - content: calculi, parasites.
- **Common bile duct:** diameter, dilated, stricture
  - *normal* – ≤6mm diameter;
  - ≤10mm post-cholecystectomy, in elderly;
  - ↑ diameter by 1mm each decade after the age of 60 years.

❶ A normal common bile duct diameter does not exclude extrahepatic obstruction:
- content: calculi, microlithiasis (sludge), parasites;
- mural lesion: carcinoma.

Pancreas
- **Pancreas:**
  - size;
  - *parenchyma* – cyst, tumour, haematoma, metastatic deposit.

- **Pancreatic duct:**
  - *diameter* – dilated, stricture;
  - *content* – calculi.
- **Peripancreatic:** fluid collections, abscess.

Spleen

- **Size:** normal: longest axis 12cm.
- Relationship to left kidney + left costal margin.
- **Parenchyma:**
  - *focal lesion* – haematoma, cyst, lymphoma, metastatic deposit, infarction;
  - *diffuse disease* – haemosiderosis.

Intraoperative ultrasound

Approach
- **Intraoperative ultrasonography** (IOUS) at open surgery using a handheld transducer on a mobile ultrasound machine (Fig. 2.1a).
- **Laparoscopic ultrasonography** (LUS): usually performed with a high resolution 7.5–10MHz probe.

Indications

Benign

Used extensively in benign biliary tract disease to identify intraductal calculi replacing the need for intraoperative chaolangiography + directing the appropriate use of laparoscopic common bile duct exploration

Malignant
- To further characterize known lesions (Fig. 2.1b,c).
- To identify additional lesions, e.g. systematic evaluation of the liver for small intraparenchymal tumours not identified on preoperative imaging.
- To clarify the relationship of a lesion to adjacent structures to plan resection.
- As a localization technique for pathology not identified on preoperative imaging studies, e.g. insulinoma.
- To facilitate intraoperative tumour biopsy.
- To optimize staging laparoscopy in pancreaticobiliary malignancy to determine unresectability + avoid unnecessary surgical intervention.
- To optimize staging laparoscopy in pancreaticobiliary malignancy to improve the sensitivity of laparoscopic staging in predicting resectability.

▶ IOUS + LUS facilitate assessment of liver metastases, local vascular involvement, and regional nodal disease.

❶ Several studies have demonstrated that LUS improves diagnostic accuracy of staging laparoscopy alone, providing additional information in 14–25% of patients.

▶ Sensitivity + specificity of intraoperative IOUS can be improved with the use of contrast agents, but their use is currently limited.

Advantages
- High accuracy.
- Rapid investigation.
- Allows real time imaging.
- Allows direct visualization of the tissue without the interference of skin, subcutaneous fat, + bowel gas.
- Low cost.
- Provides structural detail down to 1mm.
- Well tolerated procedure.
- Allows systematic evaluation of solid organs, such as the liver + pancreas with evaluation of major vascular structures.

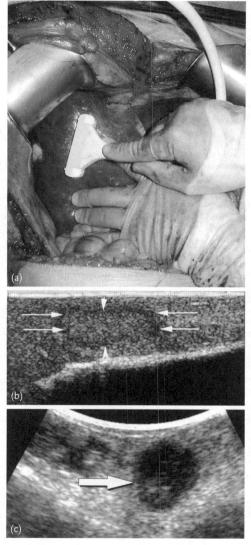

Fig. 2.1. Intraoperative ultrasound. The ultrasound probe is placed directly onto the liver (a), and allows identification of hepatic vasculature and their relationship with tumours (b and c, arrowed).

Disadvantages

- Operator dependent.
- Limited access to structures/organs in the absence of adequate organ mobilization, e.g. limited access to segments V–VIII at laparoscopy.
- Cannot be readily reviewed.
- Suboptimal quality in the obese.
- Repetition for follow-up can be difficult if performed by different operators or at wide time intervals.

The role of intraoperative ultrasonography in specific tumour types

Pancreatic adenocarcinoma

- Examination of the liver for small intraparenchymal lesions.
- Evaluation of the primary tumour's relationship to surrounding vasculature, in particular, invasion into portal vein, superior mesenteric vein or artery.
- Peripancreatic extension of tumour.

❶ Staging laparoscopy in pancreatic adenocarcinoma upstages 15–20% of patients with preoperative determined radiologically resectable disease.

❶ Staging laparoscopy with LUS provides additional data.

❶ In published reports, LUS has resulted in a change in surgical treatment in 14–36% of patients in whom standard laparoscopy was equivocal.

Other pancreatic or periampullary malignancies

- Occult metastases in non-functioning islet cell tumours.
- **Insulinoma**:
  - sensitivities of up to 95% are reported in the detection of pancreatic insulinomas using LUS;
  - the optimal resection method (i.e. enucleation or formal resection) can be determined by evaluation of tumour proximity to the main pancreatic duct, combined with colour flow Doppler assessment of adjacent major vessels.
- Prediction of resectability in periampullary non-pancreatic adenocarcinoma – duodenal, ampullary, distal bile duct tumours.

Liver tumours

- IOUS has a major impact on planned resection of primary or metastatic liver malignancies.
- IOUS has a sensitivity of 98% + specificity of 95%.
- IOUS is the gold standard for detecting liver lesions.
- IOUS is performed routinely in specialist centres prior to liver resection.
- Can accurately detect cysts of 1–3mm + solid lesions of 3–5mm diameter.

▶ Spectral + colour Doppler transducer probes should be used to assess tumour vascularity + vascular invasion.

Role of IOUS in liver malignancy

- Evaluation of extent of disease.
- Detection of occult metastases.
- Determination of respectability.

- Allows biopsy of small intraparenchymal lesions.
- Assists in surgical planning to optimize remnant liver volume, while ensuring negative margins.
- Facilitates tumour ablation, e.g. radiofrequency ablation of contralateral tumour following extended hepatectomy or with compromised parenchyma (steatohepatitis, prior liver resection) to preserve liver volume + avoid small for size syndrome.

▶ IOUS detects new findings in 40–55% of cases.

▶ IOUS changes management in 20–30% of patients.

▶ Non-R0 resection is avoided in 5% with use of IOUS.

Cross-sectional imaging

Computed tomography
- Digital processing of large number of x-ray images to generate a series of 2–5mm slices.
- Enhanced image quality using multi-slice or helical computed tomography (CT).
- Detailed anatomical resolution.
- **Limitations:** radiation exposure 10mSv (compared with average annual background radiation dose of 2.4mSv); contrast allergy; contrast-related nephropathy (iodinated contrast). In patients with renal impairment, ensure adequate hydration, consider giving IV or oral N-acetylcysteine pre-CT, or use alternative imaging (e.g. MRI).

Magnetic resonance imaging
- A magnetic field causes alignment of protons within the body and a perpendicular oscillating electromagnetic field is then applied, causing protons to rotate. Protons then emit a detectable radiofrequency signal when they revert to their original position.
- Image appearances depend on the *relaxation time*, e.g. 1s for T1-weighted images and a few milliseconds for T2-weighted images.
- IV gadolinium contrast improves sensitivity and is safer than iodinated contrast agents used in CT scanning.
- Indications in hepatobiliary disease include:
  - characterization of liver lesions (i.e. benign vs. malignant; particularly in cirrhotic livers to detect HCC);
  - staging of colorectal liver metastases;
  - evaluation of venous anatomy (magnetic resonance venography) prior to shunt surgery;
  - evaluation of pancreatic lesions.
- **Contraindications:** pacemakers, ferromagnetic implants (e.g. cochlear implants), foreign bodies.

Magnetic resonance cholangiopancreatography
- Non-invasive diagnostic technique based on MRI, which uses computer software to generate 3-D images of the biliary tree and pancreatic duct (Fig. 2.2a,b).
- **Indications:**
  - biliary obstruction, e.g. to exclude common bile duct stones;
  - evaluation of iatrogenic bile duct injury;
  - evaluation of patients after previous biliary reconstructive surgery.
- **Contraindications:** as for MRI.

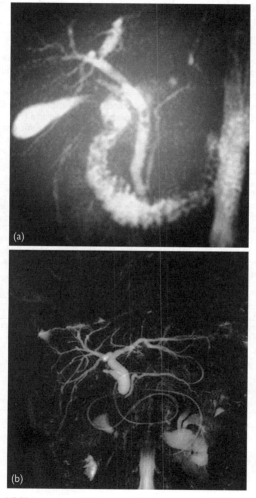

Fig. 2.2 MRCP appearances of (a) common bile duct stones and (b) hilar stricture with proximal biliary dilatation.

Hepatobiliary iminodiacetic acid scan

- Iminodiacetic acid derivatives are excreted in bile.
- Patients must be fasted for 2–24 h.
- Following IV injection of technetium-99-labelled O-dimethyl iminodiacetic acid, emitted gamma rays are detected. After a peak in hepatic activity at 20min, the common hepatic duct is visualized at 30min, and the gallbladder is seen at 30–60min. An infusion of cholecystokinin (CCK) during the scan causes increased bile flow, contraction of the gallbladder and relaxation of the sphincter of Oddi. The diagnostic accuracy of hepatobiliary iminodiacetic acid (HIDA) scans may be improved in certain conditions by using specific drugs (e.g. CCK and acalculous cholecystitis; phenobarbital and neonatal jaundice; morphine and acute cholecystitis; see Table 2.1).

Indications

- Diagnosis of acalculous cholecystitis (reduced GB ejection fraction to <35% in 20min after CCK injection).
- Diagnosis of acute calculous cholecystitis (if clinical suspicion and US not diagnostic).
- *Sphincter of Oddi dysfunction* – morphine-augmented HIDA scan may help to select patients who require ERCP and manometry.
- Post-operative bile leak (after hepatectomy or cholecystectomy).
- Detection of bile leak following blunt or penetrating liver trauma.
- Assess emptying of Roux loop if stasis suspected (see Fig. 2.3).

Table 2.1 Drugs used to improve diagnostic accuracy of HIDA scans

Drug	Action	Diagnostic use
Cholecystokinin (CCK)	Increased bile flow GB contraction Relaxation of SOD	Acalculous cholecystitis
Phenobarbital	Increased bile production (infants)	Neonatal jaundice
Morphine	Contraction of SOD	SOD dysfunction
Amyl nitrate	Increased bile flow	SOD dysfunction

SOD – sphincter of Oddi

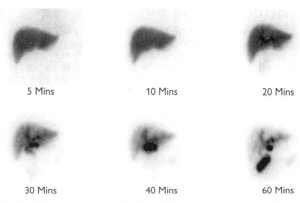

5 Mins   10 Mins   20 Mins

30 Mins   40 Mins   60 Mins

Fig. 2.3 HIDA scan in a patient with delayed biliary secretion after Roux-en-Y hepatico-jejunostomy. There is abnormal persistence of radiolabelled tracer within the Roux limb after 40min.

Positron emission tomography scan

- 2-fluoro-2-deoxy-D-glucose (FDG) is transported into cells by the glucose transporter and phosphorylated by hexokinase. It is not metabolized and therefore accumulates within cells. Tumour cells have increased rates of glycolysis and, therefore, have increased uptake of FDG. FDG-positron emission tomography (PET) scans take advantage of this process.
- Certain radio-isotopes decay by emitting positrons, which collide with electrons to emit gamma rays. Gamma rays are detected by the PET system (multiple rings of detectors containing crystals of bismuth germanium oxide or sodium iodide).
- Modern PET systems have a spatial resolution of about 5mm. Computerized data reconstruction is capable of generating a 3-D map of radioactivity. Newer systems combine CT and PET to further improve the accuracy of anatomical localization.
- PET scans are safe and highly sensitive, and are being increasingly used to improve the accuracy of preoperative staging for a range of malignant tumours.

Colorectal cancer

PET is as sensitive as CT for detecting colorectal liver metastases, but is better at detecting extra-hepatic disease (sensitivity 95%, specificity 100%).

Hepatocellular carcinoma

The role of PET for evaluating hepatocellular carcinoma (HCC) is unclear. PET is more sensitive for detecting poorly differentiated tumours, which appear 'cold' due to reducer uptake of tracer.

Cholangiocarcinoma

The role of PET is limited in patients with primary sclerosing cholangitis due to increased uptake secondary to inflammation.

Somatostatin receptor scintigraphy

- Also known as **octreotide scan**.
- IV injection of radio-labelled octreotide (a somatostatin analogue), which binds to somatostatin receptors (over-expressed by neuroendocrine tumours, e.g. carcinoid).
- Indications: diagnosis and localization of primary and metastatic neuroendocrine tumours (sensitivity of 50–80% for primary tumour and 90–95% for liver metastases).
- Improved accuracy when combined with cross-sectional imaging (CT or MRI).

Endoscopic ultrasound

Combines upper GI endoscope with integrated ultrasound probe to allow ultrasound examination of the upper GI tract, including pancreas and distal CBD. Allows US-guided fine-needle aspiration or biopsy of lesions or cysts (e.g. pancreatic cystic lesions). Endoscopic ultrasound (EUS) is an alternative to MRCP, especially for distal CBD or pancreatic pathology, and has an advantage of obtaining diagnostic cytology.

Indications

- Evaluation of suspected distal CBD stone or neoplasm.
- Assessing local extent of pancreatic cancer (e.g. nodal status and vascular encasement).
- Evaluating cystic pancreatic lesions (including aspirating fluid for cytological and biochemical analysis) for CEA and CA19.9.

Endoscopic retrograde cholangiopancreatography

Indications
- **Diagnosis:**
  - has been largely replaced by MRCP for diagnostic investigation;
  - brushings for cytology;
  - sphincter of Oddi manometry.
- **Therapeutic:**
  - stone retrieval;
  - stent placement (plastic or metallic);
  - stricture dilatation;
  - photodynamic therapy;
  - lithotripsy.

See Fig. 2.4.

Pre-procedure
- Check clotting and platelet count.
- Give IV vitamin K if patient jaundiced.
- Give prophylactic antibiotics (e.g. 750mg cefuroxime IV or 4.5g piperacillin IV) 2h before the procedure.
- Administer supplemental oxygen via nasal cannulae.
- Monitor BP, HR, SaO_2 (pulse oximetry).
- Administer sedation (IV midazolam or IV propofol). Anaesthetic input in high risk cases. Use general anaesthetic in patients with known intolerance to sedation.

Procedure
- Position patient in left lateral decubitus position.
- Insert side viewing endoscope into second part of duodenum.
- Locate and cannulate the ampulla of Vater.
- Perform sphincterotomy between 11 and 1 o'clock positions using sphincterotome.
- Retrieve stones using Dormier basket.
- Insert stent if unable to clear CBD (repeat procedure in 2–4 weeks).

Complications
- **Pancreatitis**.
- **Haemorrhage** (1%): minor bleeding is common and presents with melaena +/– haematemesis. Significant bleeding may require transfusion +/– endoscopic haemostasis (adrenaline). Surgery is rarely necessary.
- **Perforation:** localized retroperitoneal perforations in a stable patient may be managed non-operatively (NBM, IV fluids, IV antibiotics, IV omeprazole). Arrange gastrograffin swallow and/or CT with oral contrast to exclude ongoing duodenal leak. Presence of sepsis, persistent leak, or peritonitis are indications for urgent surgery.

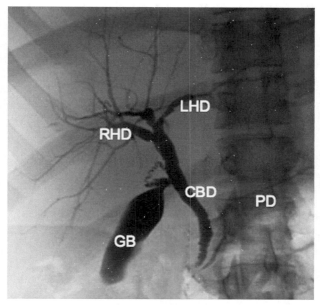

Fig. 2.4 Radiological appearance of ERCP image. RHD: right hepatic duct, LHD: left hepatic duct, CBD: common bile duct, GB: gallbladder, PD: pancreatic duct.

Percutaneous liver biopsy

Indications
- Persistently abnormal LFTs for >6 months of unknown cause.
- Histological staging of a liver disease to guide management (e.g. hepatitis C).
- Assessment of presence/severity of fibrosis of contralateral lobe prior to liver resection for malignancy.
- Allograft dysfunction post-liver transplant.
- Histological diagnosis of a liver lesion (if it will influence management).

Contraindications
- Bleeding disorders: INR>1.6; platelet count less than 60×10^9/L; unexplained bleeding; haemophilia; ascites; obesity.
- Consider alternative route of biopsy (e.g. transjugular biopsy).

Preparation
- Check FBC, INR.
- Stop NSAIDs, aspirin, and clopidogrel **1 week** before biopsy.
- Stop warfarin and give unfractionated heparin if required.
- NBM for 6h pre-procedure.

Procedure
- **Choice of needle:** *suction* (Menghini, Klatskin or Jamshidi), *cutting* (TruCut) or *spring-loaded* (Microinvasive). Larger samples with suction and cutting, **but** increased bleeding risk.
- Patient supine with right arm behind the head.
- Identify point of maximal dullness to percussion in mid-axillary line (usually 6th–8th intercostal space).
- Aseptic technique.
- Local anaesthetic infiltration.
- Ultrasound-guided approach. Used for targeted biopsy of a lesion or specific lobe. Insert needle into liver when *patient holding their breath in expiration*. A sample of 1.5cm × 1–2mm should yield 6–8 portal triads.

Post-procedure care
- 2h bed rest.
- Nursing observations every 15min for 1h, then every 30min for 1h, then hourly.

Complications
- 60% of complications occur within 2h of biopsy; 96% occur within 24h.
- Pain is common (30%). Treat with analgesia.
- Haemorrhage (subcapsular haematoma or haemoperitoneum).
- Biliary peritonitis.
- Haemobilia.
- Cholangitis.
- Sepsis.
- Visceral perforation.
- Pneumothorax.
- Mortality 0.01% (for low risk cases).

Percutaneous transhepatic cholangiography

- Puncture of intrahepatic bile duct under radiological guidance, followed by injection of iodinated contrast to generate a cholangiogram (Fig. 2.5). May be combined with percutaneous interventions, such as balloon dilatation or stent insertion.
- **Indications:**
  - investigation/management of biliary obstruction if ERCP unsuccessful or not possible (e.g. previous bilio-enteric anastomosis; previous Billroth II gastrectomy);
  - assessment of proximal bile duct involvement in patients with hilar cholangiocarcinoma;
  - investigation of recurrent cholangitis after bilio-enteric anastomosis.
- Preparation and procedure are similar to percutaneous liver biopsy (see Percutaneous liver biopsy 📖 p. 38).

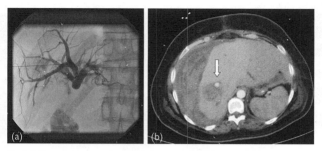

Fig. 2.5 Percutaneous transhepatic cholangiography. (a) Percutaneuous cannulation of right anterior sectoral duct demonstrating cholangiographic appearance of proximal hilar stricture. (b) The CT shows the presence of arterial injury after PTC which has led to pseudoaneurysm formation (arrow) in addition to a large subcapsular haematoma.

Perioperative care and liver disease

R. Sutcliffe

Risk assessment

- Thorough history and physical examination, particularly regarding the presence and severity of underlying liver disease and comorbidity (e.g. diabetes).
- **Assess exercise tolerance:** subjectively and/or objectively if history is suggestive (cardiopulmonary exercise testing, exercise ECG, dobutamine-stress echocardiography, thallium scan).
- **Assess severity of liver disease:** Child-Pugh or Model for End-stage Liver Disease score (MELD) (see Liver disease severity 📖 p. 64).
- Refer to cardiologist (+/– coronary angiography) if severe hypertension, poorly controlled ischaemic heart disease or symptomatic cardiac failure suspected.
- Perform baseline ABG and pulmonary function tests and/or refer to respiratory physician if symptomatic, poorly controlled asthma, COPD, or other interstitial lung disease.
- Determine ASA grade and seek anaesthetic opinion.

Preoperative management

- Ensure adequately hydrated (particularly if preoperative renal dysfunction and/or jaundice). Use IV saline and/or human albumin solution.
- Correct coagulopathy and thrombocytopaenia.
- Consider nutritional support if preoperative malnutrition.

Specific conditions

Obstructive jaundice

- 20% risk of postoperative renal failure, especially if ascending cholangitis or sepsis.
- Hyperbilirubinaemia reduces systemic vascular resistance, causes salt wasting and reduces left ventricular response to hypovolaemia. Net effect is acute renal failure due to ↑ sympathetic tone and renal vasoconstriction.
- Risk of gut bacterial translocation due to absence of protective effect of bile salts in duodenum.
- **Management:** preoperative biliary drainage (if cholangitis or preoperative renal impairment); IV antibiotics for cholangitis (piperacillin 4.5g tds or ciprofloxacin 200mg bd); fluid replacement; consider CVP monitoring; careful dosing of aminoglycosides; avoid nephrotoxic agents (e.g. NSAIDs); avoid iodinated IV contrast if possible (or supplement with N-acetylcysteine pre-imaging).

Coagulopathy

- Prolonged INR due to reduced hepatic synthesis of clotting factors and/or vitamin K deficiency (cholestasis).
- Thrombocytopaenia due to hypersplenism or sepsis.
- Replace vitamin K.
- Give fresh frozen plasma (FFP) if INR >1.5.
- Transfuse pooled platelets if platelet count $<50 \times 10^9$/L.
- Consider intraoperative thromboelastography (TEG).
- Give cryoprecipitate if fibrinogen <1.0g/L.
- Consider IV tranexamic acid (slow IV injection) 0.5–1g tds.
- Recombinant factor VII if uncontrolled coagulopathic bleeding after correction of above deficiencies.

Ascites

- Secondary to portal hypertension and hypoalbuminaemia.
- Causes splinting of diaphragm, increasing risk of respiratory complications and renal impairment.
- Increased risk of wound dehiscence and hernias.
- **Management:** leave ascitic drain *in situ* postoperatively to reduce wound complications.

Encephalopathy

- Postoperative encephalopathy has very high mortality.
- Precipitated by infection, drugs, biochemical, or metabolic disturbance, hypoxia or bleeding.
- Look for and treat the underlying cause.
- Give lactulose 20ml BD to treat/prevent constipation.
- Keep patient well hydrated.

Malnutrition

- Common in end-stage liver disease and carries high mortality.
- Hypoalbuminaemia reduces drug binding and metabolism → increased serum concentrations of anaesthetic agents, analgesics, and sedatives.
- Consider preoperative nutritional support (enteral or parenteral).
- Use high carbohydrate/lipid and reduced amino acid content to reduce risk of encephalopathy.

Ischaemic heart disease

- Significant coronary artery disease in 10% of patients with end-stage liver disease.
- Assess perioperative risk using ASA grade (Table 3.1) and Goldman cardiac risk index (Table 3.2).
- If history and/or ECG suggestive, refer for echocardiography, exercise testing, thallium scan +/– coronary angiography. Consider cardiomyopathy in alcoholic patients.

Cirrhotic cardiomyopathy

- Cirrhosis and ascites may lead to reduced left and right ventricular function.
- Mechanism? raised intra-abdominal pressure → ↑ intrathoracic pressure +/– ↑ vasoactive agents (nitric oxide, endothelin-1).
- Treatment is empirical.

Factors affecting operative risk in patients with liver disease

- Emergency > elective surgery.
- Degree of liver dysfunction (Child-Pugh or MELD scores).
- Obstructive jaundice.
- Cardiopulmonary disease.
- Renal failure.
- Type of surgery.
- Comorbidity.

Table 3.1 ASA grading system

ASA grade and definitions	Mortality (%)
(I) Normal healthy individual	0.05
(II) Mild systemic disease that does not limit activity	0.4
(III) Severe systemic disease that limits activity	4.5
(IV) Incapacitating systemic disease which is constantly life-threatening	25
(V) Moribund not expected to survive 24h	50

Table 3.2 Goldman cardiac risk index

Third heart sound (S3)	11
Elevated JVP	11
Recent MI (<6 months)	10
ECG: premature atrial contraction	7
ECG: >5 ventricular ectopics per min	7
Age >70 years	5
Emergency procedure	4
Thoracic or abdominal surgery	3
Poor general status	3
Goldman score	**Mortality**
>25	56%
<25	4%
<6	0.2%

Hepatopulmonary syndrome

- Develops in up to 15% of patients with end-stage liver disease.
- Definition = hypoxaemia + R–L shunt + increased A–a gradient in absence of cardiopulmonary disease.

   A–a gradient = $(FiO_2\%/100) \times [(Patm - 47mmHg) - (PaCO_2/0.8) - PaO_2]$

- Characterized by:
  - pulmonary hypertension;
  - systemic-to-pulmonary shunting;
  - intrapulmonary shunting leading to arterial hypoxaemia.
- Treatment is by liver transplantation.

Hepatorenal syndrome

- **Definition:** renal failure in cirrhosis in the absence of definable cause (e.g. sepsis, drugs).
- Pathogenesis unknown.
- **Pathology:** imbalance between vasodilators (PGE_2) and vasoconstrictors (renin-angiotensin system, endothelin) $\Rightarrow$ renal cortical vasoconstriction $\Rightarrow$ renal failure.
- **Type I:** rapidly progressive, high mortality.
- **Type II:** moderate reduction in GFR. Treat by reducing portal hypertension (e.g. terlipressin). Avoid nephrotoxins, adequate fluid replacement, treat infections.

Portopulmonary hypertension

- 10% patients with end-stage liver disease.
- **Definition:** portal hypertension + mean PAP >25mmHg in absence of heart failure (PCWP <15mmHg).
- **Pathogenesis:** pulmonary vasoconstriction and thrombosis.
- If severe (PAP > 45), mortality after liver transplant is nearly 100%.
- Treatment options are limited. Consider nebulized prostacyclin or trial of sildenafil.

Anaesthetic considerations

Liver disease and general anaesthesia
- Hypoalbuminaemia reduces drug binding and metabolism resulting in increased serum concentrations.
- Patients with liver disease have a reduced catecholamine response and have impaired ability to compensate for hypovolaemia.
- Anaesthetic agents (especially halothane and enflurane) cause systemic vasodilatation and negative inotropic effects, leading to reduced hepatic blood flow and deterioration in liver function.
- Halothane also directly hepatotoxic. Isoflurane is safe and may increase hepatic blood flow. Propofol is a useful induction agent.
- Avoid or use reduced dose of drugs that are metabolized by liver/kidneys (e.g. opioids, benzodiazepines, barbiturates). Remifentanil is metabolized by tissue and red cell esterases, and is the opioid of choice.
- The preferred neuromuscular blocking agent is atracurium.

Reperfusion syndrome
- Characterized by acute haemodynamic instability and/or acute lung injury developing after reperfusion of a transplanted liver.
- Exacerbated by massive transfusion.
- Treatment is supportive (cardiorespiratory support).

Type of surgery
- **Abdominal surgery:** traction on abdominal viscera causes reflex hypotension + reduced hepatic blood flow.
- **Laparoscopy:** laparoscopic cholecystectomy is safe in patients with compensated liver disease (Child A or B) without portal hypertension (varices).
- **Previous surgery:** increased risk of intraoperative blood loss, exacerbated by portal hypertension and coagulopathy.
- **Liver resection:** high mortality in patients with chronic liver disease (9%) and obstructive jaundice (21%).
- **Emergency surgery:** high mortality compared with elective surgery. Related to Child-Pugh score and severity of portal hypertension.

Intraoperative monitoring
- All patients should have invasive monitoring (arterial and CVP).
- Internal jugular vein is preferred route in patients with coagulopathy.
- For patients with severe liver disease undergoing major surgery, fluid/inotrope therapy should be guided by either transoesophageal echocardiography (TOE), pulmonary artery catheter (PAC) or pulse contour cardiac output (PiCCO).
- **Thromboelastography:** rapid, real-time intraoperative assessment of global thrombodynamic properties of blood. Measures kinetics, strength, and stability of clot formation. Impaired clotting must be corrected with FFP, platelets, and cryoprecipitate as indicated.

Postoperative analgesia
- IV morphine PCA is preferred.
- Intramuscular injection and epidural analgesia are contraindicated in coagulopathic patients.

Parenchymal liver disease

C. Antoniades, N. Philips, R. Sutcliffe, & O. Tucker

Symptoms and signs of liver disease

Symptoms
- **Non-specific:** malaise, gastrointestinal symptoms, anorexia/weight loss.
- **Haematemesis or melaena:** oesophageal varices, peptic ulcer/gastritis.
- **Abdominal pain or discomfort:** due to hepatomegaly, hepatitis, hepatic malignancy, cholangitis, gallstones, ascites, spontaneous bacterial peritonitis.
- **Jaundice:** yellowish discoloration of sclerae or skin. Serum bilirubin >45µmol/L. Pale stools and dark urine suggests extrahepatic bile duct obstruction. Associated with pruritus due to cholestasis.
- **Dyspnoea:** due to fluid retention, ascites.
- **Spontaneous bleeding:** due to clotting factor deficiency and/or thrombocytopaenia.
- **Encephalopathy:** sleep disturbance, loss of higher cortical functions, altered personality, drowsiness, confusion, coma.

History
- Previous blood transfusion.
- Recent foreign travel.
- Previous jaundice.
- Sexual contacts.
- Drug history.

Jaundice: causes
Unconjugated
- Over-production of bilirubin due to haemolysis.
- Impaired hepatic bilirubin uptake.
- Inherited defects of conjugation (Gilberts, Criglar Najjar).

Conjugated
- Extrahepatic biliary obstruction (cholelithiasis, cholangiocarcinoma, biliary strictures, pancreatic cancer).
- Intrahepatic cholestasis (hepatitis A/B/C, CMV, EBV, alcoholic, non-alcoholic, drug-induced, primary sclerosing cholangitis).
- Failure to excrete conjugated bilirubin (Dubin-Johnson syndrome).

Hepatic encephalopathy grading (Table 4.1)

Table 4.1 Hepatic encephalopathy grading

Grade	
1	Alert, depressed, poor concentration
2	Drowsy, lethargic, disorientation
3	Very drowsy, but rousable, marked confusion, incoherent speech, flapping tremor
4	Coma, unresponsive

Hepatic encephalopathy: precipitating factors
- Constipation.
- Protein meal.

- Gastrointestinal bleed.
- Dehydration.
- Electrolyte disturbance.
- Metabolic disturbance.
- Infection.
- Drugs.

Signs

General

- Signs of malnutrition, e.g. muscle wasting, thinning of skin.
- Jaundice.
- Hyperpigmentation (PBC, haemochromatosis).
- Vitiligo (associated with autoimmune diseases, e.g. PBC, CAH).
- Excoriations (secondary to scratching seen with pruritus).
- Bruising.
- Gynaecomastia.

Face

- Kayser-Fleischer rings (greenish-blue deposition of copper pigment in Descemet's membrane near posterior surface of cornea) present in 90% of patients with neurological manifestations of Wilson's disease.
- Spider naevi. More than three suggests chronic liver disease.

Hands

- Palmar erythema (red discoloration affecting thenar and hypothenar eminences) associated with liver disease, rheumatoid arthritis, thyrotoxicosis, and pregnancy.
- Dupuytren's contracture (thickening of palmar fascia causing flexion contractures of the fingers) is associated with alcohol consumption, rather than liver disease.
- Leukonychia (white nails due to hypoalbuminaemia).
- Finger clubbing.

Cardiovascular/respiratory

- **Cardiomyopathy:** alcohol-related liver disease and haemochromatosis.
- High cardiac output/low systemic vascular resistance state (warm peripheries, bounding pulse, tachycardia).
- **Hepatopulmonary syndrome:** dyspnoea, pleural effusion.

Abdomen

- Ascites (portal hypertension, portal vein thrombosis, spontaneous bacterial peritonitis, malignancy).
- Visible abdominal wall veins, including caput medusae (portal hypertension).
- Splenomegaly (portal hypertension; see Table 4.2 for other causes).
- Hepatomegaly (see Table 4.3 for causes).

Encephalopathy

Mild to severe reduction in conscious level and/or cognitive function.

Table 4.2 Splenomegaly: causes

Infection	Glandular fever
	Epstein-Barr virus
	Malaria
	Kala-Azar
	Schistosomiasis
	Tuberculosis
Congestion	Cirrhosis
	Portal or splenic vein thrombosis
	Veno-occlusive disease
	Cardiac failure
Haematological	Leukaemia
	Lymphoma
	Myeloproliferative disorders
	Haemolytic anaemia
	Idiopathic thrombocytopaenic purpura
Other	Bacterial endocarditis
	Infarction
	Felty's syndrome

Table 4.3 Hepatomegaly: causes

Congenital	Riedl's lobe
	Polycystic liver disease
	Cirrhosis (Wilson's, α1-antitrypsin deficiency, Gaucher's disease)
Acquired	Hepatitis (alcoholic, viral, autoimmune, drugs)
	Cirrhosis (alcohol, viral, PBC, PSC, secondary biliary cirrhosis)
	Tumour (hepatocellular carcinoma, cholangiocarcinoma, metastases)
	Infiltration (amyloid, sarcoid, leukaemia)
	Infection (amoebic liver abscess, schistosomiasis, hydatid cyst)
	Congestion (Budd-Chiari syndrome, congestive cardiac failure)

Acute liver failure

Definitions

Fulminant hepatic failure
Outdated term used to describe patients who develop hepatic encephalopathy within 8 weeks of the onset of symptoms, in the absence of previous liver disease.

Hyperacute liver failure
Jaundice to encephalopathy time <7 days (in the absence of pre-existing liver disease).

Acute liver failure
Jaundice to encephalopathy time 8–28 days (in the absence of pre-existing liver disease).

Subacute liver failure
Jaundice to encephalopathy time 5–26 weeks (in the absence of pre-existing liver disease).

Causes

Drugs
- Paracetamol.
- Ecstasy (methylenedioxymethamphetamine, MDMA).
- Isoniazid.
- Halothane.
- Rifampicin.
- Statins.
- NSAIDs.

Infections
- Hepatitis A.
- Hepatitis B.
- Hepatitis D.
- Hepatitis E.
- Seronegative hepatitis.

Miscellaneous
- Acute Wilson's disease.
- Acute Budd-Chiari syndrome.
- Acute fatty liver of pregnancy.
- HELLP syndrome (Haemolysis, Elevated Liver enzymes and Low Platelets) in pregnant women with pre-eclampsia or eclampsia.
- Malignant infiltration (e.g. lymphoma).
- Ischaemic hepatitis.
- Autoimmune hepatitis.
- Amanita phalloides (mushroom poisoning).

Clinical presentation
- Progressive jaundice.
- Hepatic encephalopathy. In hyperacute liver failure, grade IV encephalopathy is associated with significant cerebral oedema

and intracranial hypertension. Severe uncontrolled intracranial hypertension may lead to brainstem herniation, which is the mode of death in a significant group of patients.
- Systemic vasodilatation and shock.
- ARDS.
- **Renal failure:** paracetamol is directly nephrotoxic and contributes to acute renal failure in 75% of patients.
- Coagulopathy.
- Lactic acidosis.
- Hypoglycaemia.
- Haemolytic anaemia (Wilson's disease).
- Impaired immunity (risk of secondary infections).

Prognosis
- Depends on aetiology.
- Survival in patients with grade 3 or 4 encephalopathy:
  - *paracetamol* – 56%;
  - *hepatitis A* – 67%;
  - *hepatitis B* – 38%;
  - *seronegative* – 20%;
  - *Wilson's disease* – 1%;
  - *pregnancy-related* – 98%.
- King's College Hospital criteria for paracetamol and non-paracetamol aetiologies are widely used (see Tables 4.4 and 4.5).
- Clichy criteria. Based on a series of patients with acute liver failure (ALF) due to hepatitis B (see Acute liver failure, Clichy criteria 📖 p. 60). Used in northern Europe.

Management
Medical care
- Early referral to liver transplant unit.
- Assess prognosis (see Acute liver failure, Prognosis 📖 p. 59) +/– list for superurgent liver transplantation.
- Start N-acetylcysteine infusion (loading dose 150mg/kg then 100mg/kg continuous infusion). Reduces mortality in paracetamol-induced ALF and may also be beneficial in non-paracetamol aetiologies.
- Invasive monitoring in HDU/ITU.
- Treat organ failure as indicated:
  - mechanical ventilation;
  - haemofiltration;
  - vasopressors/inotropes.
- Prophylactic antibiotics and antifungals.
- Acid suppression.
- Monitor jugular bulb SjO_2 (reverse jugular line) to guide management of intracranial hypertension.
- Insert ICP monitor if grade IV encephalopathy/cerebral oedema.
- Do not correct coagulopathy, unless required for invasive procedures (e.g. ICP monitor or liver transplant), since INR is an important prognostic marker.

Table 4.4 King's College Hospital prognostic criteria: paracetamol-induced acute liver failure

Parameter	Sensitivity	Specificity	Positive predictive value
pH < 7.30	49%	99%	81%
All of the following at the same time:	45%	94%	67%
(1) INR > 6.5			
(2) Creatinine > 300 μmol/L			
(3) Grade 3–4 encephalopathy			

O'Grady JG, Alexander GJ, Hayllar KM, Williams R. Early indicators of prognosis in fulminant hepatic failure. *Gastroenterology* 1989; 97(2): 439–45.

Table 4.5 King's College Hospital prognostic criteria: non-paracetamol-induced acute liver failure

Parameter	Sensitivity	Specificity	Positive predictive value
INR >6.7	34%	100%	46%
Any 3 of the following:	93%	90%	92%
(1) Aetiology seronegative of autoimmune			
(2) Age <10 or >40 years			
(3) Acute or subacute			
(4) Bilirubin >300 μmol/L			
(5) INR >3.5			

Clichy criteria

Transplant if:
- Grade III or IV encephalopathy.
- Factor V < 20% (if <30 years).
- Factor V < 30% (if >30 years).

Intracranial hypertension

Cerebral perfusion pressure (CPP) =

Mean arterial pressure (MAP) – Intracranial pressure (ICP)

Maintain CPP >70 mmHg.
- Maintain MAP by adequate volume loading and/or inotropes as guided by CVP or cardiac output measurements.
- Reduce ICP:
  - nurse patient 15° head up;
  - mild hypothermia (temperature 35.5–36°C);

- high/normal serum sodium (145–150mmol/L), with strong sodium infusion – treat diabetes insipidus using DDAVP;
- bolus mannitol 1.5g/kg if oculomotor nerve (third cranial nerve) palsy (suggesting tentorial herniation) – can be repeated until serum osmolality >320;
- intermittent periods of mild hyperventilation to achieve $PaCO_2$ 4.5–5.0kPa – may be used intermittently for ICP surges, but is detrimental if prolonged due to its effect on cerebral vasoconstriction.

Liver support devices
- Bioartificial liver and extracorporeal liver assist devices (ELAD) have been tested in clinical studies as a potential bridge to liver transplantation, and lead to biochemical, but not clinical improvement.
- *Ex vivo* perfusion using pig or marginal human livers has also been tested in small studies, but its role remains unclear.
- Hepatocyte transplantation. Isolation, purification, and culture of human hepatocytes, which are then infused into the portal vein. Not currently established as an effective technique in acute liver failure.

Liver transplantation
- Currently the only effective treatment of patients with acute liver failure who have a poor prognosis according to King's College criteria.
- Acute liver failure is prioritized as 'superurgent' in the UK (category 1 in USA).
- Majority of patients with ALF who fulfil transplant criteria in the UK should receive an organ within 48h.
- The major challenge is to allocate organs only to patients who are unlikely to recover spontaneously (i.e. medical therapy alone).
- Patients should be identified sufficiently early in their disease course before serious complications develop (e.g. refractory intracranial hypertension or sepsis) that might render them untransplantable.
- Surges in ICP are common during reperfusion and may persist for 12–24h post-transplant.
- Auxiliary liver transplantation (see Auxiliary liver transplantation ☐ p. 116) is an option for patients who have the potential to recover normal liver function.
- Factors that affect outcome after transplantation include:
  - *age* – worse survival for patients >60 years;
  - *aetiology* (see Acute liver failure, Causes ☐ p. 58);
  - *renal failure*.

Cirrhosis

Causes
- Alcohol.
- Viral hepatitis (hepatitis B, hepatitis C).
- Primary biliary cirrhosis.
- Primary sclerosing cholangitis.
- Haemochromatosis.
- Autoimmune hepatitis.
- Wilson's disease.
- Non-alcoholic steatohepatitis (NASH).
- Non-alcoholic fatty liver disease (NAFLD).

Initial investigations
- FBC, reticulocyte count, Coomb's test, blood film.
- Clotting, albumin (synthetic function).
- Renal function (hepatorenal syndrome).
- Glucose (haemochromatosis/pancreatic disease).
- Liver function tests. ALT >1000IU/L suggests acute hepatic damage secondary to viral hepatitis, ischaemia, or medications. Raised ALP and GGT suggest biliary obstruction.
- **Virology:** hepatitis A/B/C, EBV, CMV.
- Alpha-foetoprotein (hepatocellular carcinoma).
- CA-19.9 (cholangiocarcinoma).
- Iron studies (including ferritin).
- **Autoantibodies:** anti-nuclear antibody, anti-mitochondrial antibody, anti-liver kidney smooth muscle antibody.
- Immunoglobulins.
- Copper and caeruloplasmin (Wilson's disease).
- Culture urine, blood, ascitic fluid.
- **Urine:** lack of bilirubin in the context of jaundice indicates unconjugated hyperbilirubinaemia.
- **CXR**: pleural effusions, malignancy.
- **Ultrasound:** biliary dilatation, gallstones, pancreatic mass, hepatic lesions, splenomegaly.

Management of cirrhosis
Principles
- Slow/reverse liver disease.
- Prevent further damage.
- Prevent/treat complications.
- Appropriate selection of patients for liver transplantation.

General approach
- Establish diagnosis.
- Investigate for underlying cause.
- Assess severity (Child-Pugh score or MELD).
- Abstain from alcohol.
- Avoid hepatotoxic drugs.
- Vaccinate against hepatitis A/B.
- Prophylactic antibiotics if previous spontaneous bacterial peritonitis.

- Screening upper GI endoscopy. Medical/endoscopic therapy for oesophageal varices (see Portal hypertension 📖 p. 66).
- Surveillance for hepatocellular carcinoma (serum AFP and USS every 6 months). High risk groups – HBV, HCV, haemochromatosis, alcoholic cirrhosis, PBC. (see Hepatocellular carcinoma 📖 p. 150).
- Disease-specific therapies, e.g. PEG interferon and ribavirin for HCV, steroids/immunosuppression for autoimmune hepatitis.

Nutritional assessment

- Protein energy malnutrition common in cirrhosis.
- Reduced intake due to encephalopathy, unpalatable low sodium diet, nausea, anorexia.
- Impaired digestion due to intestinal dysmotility, bacterial overgrowth, bile salt malabsorption.
- Abnormal metabolism. Preferential metabolism of fat, ↓ gluconeogenesis and ↓ glycogen storage, ↓ protein absorption, ↓ hepatic protein synthesis, ↑ urinary nitrogen excretion. Catabolic state during decompensation.
- Management includes assessment by dietician, daily weights, food diary, history of gastritis/diarrhoea, assessment of severity of cirrhosis, fat soluble vitamins (A D E K), vitamin C, B12, thiamine, folate, zinc.

Liver disease severity

Child-Pugh score
- Proposed by C.G. Child and J.G. Turcotte in 1964 (University of Michigan). Modified by Pugh in 1972.
- Also known as Child-Turcotte-Pugh classification.
- Incorporates five variables: bilirubin, ascites, INR, encephalopathy, serum albumin.
- Measure of severity of chronic liver disease (see Tables 4.6 and 4.7).
- Indicator of prognosis.

Table 4.6 Calculating Child-Pugh score

Variable	Score		
	1	2	3
Bilirubin µmol/l	<34	34–51	>51
Ascites	Absent	Slight	Moderate
INR	<1.3	1.3–1.5	>1.5
Albumin g/l	>35	28–35	<28
Encephalopathy	Grade 0	Grade 1–2	Grade 3–4

INR = international normalized ratio

Table 4.7 Child-Pugh classification

	Score	1-year survival (%)
A – well compensated	5–6	100
B – significant functional compromise	7–9	80
C – decompensated	10–15	45

Model for End-stage Liver Disease (MELD)
Originally developed to assess the prognosis of cirrhotic patients undergoing TIPS. Now used in USA and Europe to stratify patients on waiting list for liver transplantation. Equivalent to the Child-Pugh score in a non-transplant setting.

Calculated by the following equation:

$$\text{MELD} = [3.78 \times \log_e(\text{plasma bilirubin})] + [11.2 \times \log_e(\text{INR})] + [9.57 \times \log_e(\text{plasma creatinine})] + 6.43$$

- Paediatric version (PELD) also available.
- Online MELD and PELD calculator available at UNOS website (www.unos.org/resources/meldPeldCalculator.asp).

UK Model for End-stage Liver Disease (UKELD)
- Developed from analysis of 1103 patients.
- UKELD score >49 predicts 1-year mortality >9%. Used as minimum listing criteria for liver transplantation in UK.

Further information

Child, C.G., & Turcotte, J.G. (1964) Surgery and portal hypertension. In: C.G. Child (Ed.) The liver and portal hypertension. Saunders, Philadelphia: 50–64.

Kamath, P.S., Wiesner, R.H., Malinchoc, M., Kremers, W., Therneau, T.M., Kosberg, C.L., D'Amico, G., Dickson, E.R., & Kim, W.R. (2001) A model to predict survival in patients with end-stage liver disease. *Hepatology* **33**, 464–70.

Pugh, R.N., Murray-Lyon, I.M., Dawson, J.L., Pietroni, M.C., & Williams, R. (1973) Transection of the oesophagus for bleeding oesophageal varices. *Br J Surg* **60**(8), 646–9.

Portal hypertension

- PV-IVC pressure gradient >12mmHg.
- Development of collateral vessels (varices) at sites of portosystemic anastomoses (gastro-oesophageal junction, rectum, left renal vein, retroperitoneum, anterior abdominal wall, diaphragm).
- Associated with splenomegaly, ascites, and encephalopathy.

Causes

Prehepatic

- Portal vein thrombosis (idiopathic in 30%).
- Splenic vein thrombosis (segmental or left-sided portal hypertension).
- Extrinsic compression of portal vein.
- Congenital atresia or stenosis of portal vein.

Intrahepatic

- Cirrhosis.
- Schistosomiasis.
- Hepatic metastases.
- Infiltration by haematological diseases.
- Polycystic disease.
- Granulamatous disease – sarcoid and TB.
- Amyloidosis.
- Acute alcoholic hepatitis.
- Hepatocellular carcinoma.
- Non-cirrhotic portal hypertension.
- Vitamin A toxicity.
- Chemical toxicity – arsenic, vinyl chloride, copper sulphate.
- Congenital hepatic fibrosis.
- Nodular reactive hyperplasia.
- Rendu-Osler-Weber syndrome.
- Acute fatty liver of pregnancy.

Post-hepatic

- Hepatic vein thrombosis (Budd-Chiari syndrome).
- Veno-occlusive disease (bone marrow transplant, chemotherapy).
- Constrictive pericarditis.
- Right heart failure (tricuspid valve abnormalities).

Pathophysiology

- **Increased vascular resistance:** cirrhosis → architectural distortion + stellate cell activation → ↑ vascular resistance → increased portal pressure (Poiseuille's law).
- **Increased portal blood flow:** cirrhosis → peripheral + splanchnic vasodilatation (mediated by glucagon, nitric acid, ANP, prostaglandins) → relative hypovolaemia → renin-angiotensin system activation → salt/water retention → increased portal blood flow → further increase in portal pressure.

Clinical features

- Asymptomatic.
- Variceal bleeding (haematemesis/melaena).

- Ascites (distension, dyspnoea due to diaphragmatic splinting).
- Spontaneous bacterial peritonitis (abdominal pain and fever).
- Encephalopathy (irritability, altered sleep patterns, poor memory, and confusion).
- Splenomegaly.
- Caput medusae.

Investigations
- Investigate cause of cirrhosis.
- **US/CT:** ascites, splenomegaly, portal or splenic vein thrombosis.
- Hepatic venous pressure gradient (HVPG).
- **Upper GI endoscopy:** screening/treatment of oesophageal varices.
- Liver biopsy.

Management
Medical options
- Low sodium diet.
- Abstinence from alcohol.
- Treat underlying liver disease.
- Non-selective beta-blockers.
- Spironolactone.
- Vasopressin.
- Somatostatin analogues.
- Angiogenesis inhibitors (VEGF antagonists).

Endoscopic options
- **Endoscopic band ligation:** primary prevention if contraindication or intolerance to beta-blockers; secondary prevention (prevent rebleeding); treatment of acute bleeding.
- **Sengstaken-Blakemore tube** (if failed endoscopic therapy of acute bleed).

Interventional radiology
Transjugular intrahepatic portosytemic shunt (TIPS). After cannulating the internal jugular vein, a guide wire is passed into the right hepatic vein, and a stent inserted between RHV and portal vein. Complications include stent migration/occlusion, rebleeding (20% at 2 years), encephalopathy, hepatic decompensation. Contraindicated in severe liver disease (Child-Pugh class C or MELD score >18) and hepatic encephalopathy.

Surgical options
- Portosystemic shunt (Fig. 4.1).
- Devascularization procedures: gastroesophageal devascularization, oesophageal transaction, and splenectomy.
- Liver transplantation.

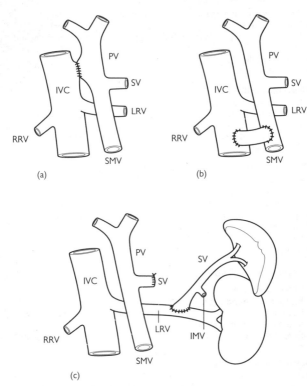

Fig. 4.1 Portosystemic shunts. (a) Side-to-side portocaval shunt. (b) Mesocaval shunt. (c) Distal spleno-renal shunt. IVC: inferior vena cava, RRV: right renal vein, LRV: left renal vein, PV: portal vein, SV: splenic vein, SMV: superior mesenteric vein, IMV: inferior mesenteric vein.

Oesophageal varices

Risk factors for bleeding
- Diameter of varix.
- Endoscopic red signs (red whale markings, cherry red spots).
- Child-Pugh score.
- Active alcohol intake in ALD.

Endoscopic grading
- **Grade 1:** small, straight.
- **Grade 2:** tortuous <1/3 lumen.
- **Grade 3:** coil shaped >1/3 lumen.

Primary prevention
- **Non-selective beta-blockers** (propanolol 40–80mg bd): titrate dose to HR 60bpm. Reduces risk of index bleed by 50%. Side effects include bronchospasm, impotence.
- **Endoscopic variceal band ligation** (VBL): indicated if intolerance or contraindications to beta-blocker. Repeat endoscopy at 3 months and annually.

Acute variceal bleeding
- Make rapid assessment of ABC.
- Call anaesthetist to secure airway (to prevent aspiration) if reduced conscious level or large volume haematemesis.
- Large bore IV cannula.
- Correct coagulopathy with FFP +/– platelet transfusion.
- Transfuse packed red blood cells if active bleeding and patient hypovolaemic.
- Send cultures and start broad spectrum antibiotics (e.g. piperacillin 4.5g tds).
- Give IV terlipressin 1mg and continue 1–2mg qds for 72h.
- Upper GI endoscopy when stable – injection sclerotherapy or variceal band ligation.
- Balloon tamponade with Sengstaken-Blakemore tube (see p. 71) if endoscopic haemostasis fails.
- Consider TIPS if endoscopic control fails.
- **Risk factors for early rebleed** (within 6 weeks): age >60 years, severe liver disease, renal failure, haemodynamic instability, ascites, active bleeding at endoscopy, Grade 3 varices with red signs. 50% of early rebleeds occur within 48h.

Secondary prevention
- 70% risk of rebleed within 1 year of index bleed.
- 30% risk of mortality with each episode.
- Variceal band ligation and beta-blockers.
- Consider portosystemic shunt surgery if portal vein occluded.
- Liver transplantation.

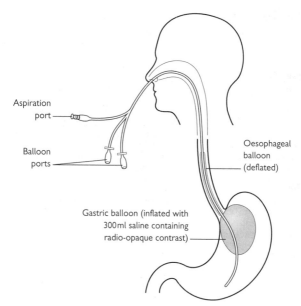

Fig. 4.2 Sengstaken-Blakemore tube. After inserting the tube into the stomach, the gastric balloon should be inflated with 300mL of saline containing radio-opaque contrast (e.g. Omnipaque) to allow radiological confirmation of position. Traction is applied by securely taping the tube to the side of the patient's face. The oesophageal balloon should not be inflated as this may cause mucosal ischaemia and exacerbate variceal bleeding.

Ascites

- 60% of patients with cirrhosis will develop ascites in 10 years.
- 5% of patients have a second cause in addition to cirrhosis, e.g. diabetic nephropathy, cardiac failure, malignancy, TB.

Investigations

- **Duplex ultrasound:** assess patency of portal vein, presence of liver lesions (e.g. HCC).
- **Ascitic tap:** aseptic technique in LIF. Fluid appearance – straw-coloured (uncomplicated), turbid (infection), milky (chylous ?malignancy), bloody (traumatic). Send fluid for cell count, albumin, protein, culture, LDH, glucose, amylase, TB smear and cytology.
- Serum/ascites albumin gradient (SAAG) = serum (albumin) – ascitic (albumin). Portal hypertension if SAAG >11g/L (97% accurate).

Management

- Aim to reduce ascites and peripheral oedema without causing intravascular volume depletion. Relieves symptoms, but does not affect patient survival.
- Abstain from alcohol.
- Low salt diet (<2g/day).
- Avoid NSAIDs.
- Maintain serum [K] >3.4 mmol/L
- Diuretics.
- Paracentesis (see Fig. 4.3).

Diuretic therapy

- **Mechanism:** improved sodium excretion.
- Aim for maximum weight loss 0.5kg/day (>0.5kg/day causes hypovolaemia).
- **Spironolactone** (aldosterone antagonist): starting dose 50–100mg od. Maximum dose 400mg od. Side effects include gynaecomastia, hyperkalaemia.
- **Frusemide** (loop diuretic): starting dose 40mg od. Use in combination with spironolactone if [K] normal/high. Use instead of spironolactone if [K} low.
- Monitor for clinical effect and check electrolytes.
- **Diuretic-resistant ascites:** occurs in 10%. Exclude HCC, PV thrombosis. Poor survival (25% at 1 year).

Paracentesis

- Treatment of large volume diuretic-resistant ascites.
- If removing >5L, give IV 20% human albumin solution (HAS) 100ml for every 2L. Can be repeated every 2 weeks, whilst awaiting definitive treatment (TIPS or liver transplantation).

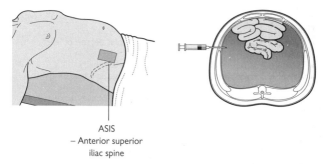

ASIS
— Anterior superior
iliac spine

Fig. 4.3 Abdominal paracentesis. The patient is positioned supine, and the left or right iliac fossa is cleaned with antiseptic solution. After percussion to confirm dullness, local anaesthetic is infiltrated just anterior to the anterior superior iliac spine (ASIS). Aspiration of straw coloured fluid confirms entry into the peritoneal cavity. A drain is then inserted using the Seldinger technique and secured in position. Paracentesis should be performed under ultrasound guidance in patients who have had previous abdominal surgery, or if previous attempts have failed.

Alcohol-related liver disease

General
- Quantity of alcohol consumed does not predict degree of liver damage.
- Women and South Asians have increased susceptibility.
- **Genetic component:** 3× the risk in monozygotic compared with dizygotic twins.
- Alcohol accelerates liver injury associated with obesity, toxins, and hepatitis C.

Fatty liver
- Alcohol metabolized by the liver results in production of nicotinamide adenine dinucleotide (NADH), which leads to accumulation of triglycerides.
- **Causes:** obesity, diabetes, and alcohol.
- **Clinical features:** often asymptomatic.
- **Diagnosis:** usually made by US performed for investigation of abnormal LFTs.
- **Management:** advice to abstain from alcohol (fatty change is reversible).
- **Liver biopsy** should be performed to confirm and stage the disease in high risk patients (age >45, coexistent hypertension, BMI >30, type 2 diabetes, hypercholesterolaemia) and those who show no improvement in LFTS after 2 months of abstinence from alcohol.

Alcoholic hepatitis
- Develops on a background of cirrhosis if consumption >80g/day of alcohol.
- **Pathology:** active inflammation with neutrophil infiltrate, focal necrosis, and hepatocyte ballooning.
- **Clinical features:** signs of alcohol withdrawal (tremor, agitation, tachycardia), jaundice, fever, palpable tender hepatomegaly.
- AST>ALT (AST = 2 × ULN).
- **Modified Maddrey discriminant function** predicts outcome.

  Discriminant function = 4.6 × (prothrombin time minus control, in s) + serum bilirubin (µmol/L)/17.

If score >32, start trial of steroids (prednisolone 40mg od) followed by tapering dose (reduces mortality from 65% to 20% at 1 month). Fall in bilirubin at 1 week predicts improved survival.
- If discriminant function score >54 response to treatment likely to be extremely poor.

Alcoholic cirrhosis
- 5-year survival depends on continued drinking (30%) vs. abstinence (70%).
- **Pathology:** micronodular cirrhosis.
- **Management:** aims are
  - treat withdrawal;
  - achieve long-term abstinence;

- treat complications of cirrhosis (ascites, varices, encephalopathy);
- surveillance for hepatocellular carcinoma (US and serum alpha-foetoprotein every 6 months).
- **Alcohol withdrawal:** reducing dose of chlordiazepoxide (start at 20mg qds); Pabrinex; multivitamins; oral thiamine; IV lorazepam for seizures; check haematinics; assess for Wernicke's encephalopathy (confusion, nystagmus, cranial nerve VI palsy, ataxia, Korsakoff's psychosis – short-term memory loss and confabulation). Emergency treatment with high dose thiamine.

Viral hepatitis

Causes
- Hepatitis A.
- Hepatitis B.
- Hepatitis C.
- Delta virus.
- Hepatitis E.
- Cytomegalovirus (CMV).
- Epstein-Barr virus (EBV).
- Herpes simplex.

Clinical features
- **History:** prodromal illness (2 days–2 weeks) – malaise, anorexia, fever, myalgia. Jaundice develops as symptoms resolve.
- **Acute hepatitis B:** arthritis, urticarial rash, membranous glomerulonephritis.
- **Hepatitis C:** cryoglobulin-induced glomerulonephritis.
- **Examination:** Jaundice; tender hepatomegaly; splenomegaly (EBV); lymphadenopathy (EBV).

Investigations
- LFTs: AST >10× upper limit of normal indicates acute hepatitis.
- **Monospot. FBC and blood film:** atypical lymphocytes (EBV and CMV).
- CMV PCR.
- Hepatitis A IgM.
- **HBsAg:** if positive, test for HBeAg (infectivity) and anti-HDV (co-infection).
- **HCV Ab:** if positive, test genotype and viral load.

Hepatitis A
- Faecal-oral transmission.
- 6 weeks incubation.
- Endemic in Middle east and Asia.
- Anti-HAV IgM positivity indicates infection in last 8 weeks.
- Anti-HAV IgG develops within 2 weeks of infection, persist for years.
- No carrier or chronic infection occurs.

Hepatitis B
- Blood-borne and sexually transmitted.
- 4–26 weeks incubation.
- **High-risk groups:** intravenous drug users (IVDU), homosexuals, neonates of HBV +ive mothers.
- HBsAg +ive for more than 6 months = carrier status.
- 5–20% develop chronic disease.
- Approx 1% will develop HBsAb per year.
- **Chronic disease:** if mild inflammation on biopsy no treatment needed.
- If HBeAg +ive and viral load is high (HBV DNA >10^5 copies per mL) with inflammation on liver biopsy, consider antiviral treatment.

Hepatitis C

- Blood-borne and sexually transmitted.
- 6–12-week incubation.
- **High-risk groups:** IVDU, transfusions, haemophiliacs.
- Carrier state exists and 70% develop chronic infection.
- Up to 20% develop cirrhosis within 20 years of infection.
- If HCV Ab +ive, test PCR RNA load (increased within 6 weeks of acute infection) and hepatitis C genotype (type 2/3 has a better response than type 1) to predict response to treatment.
- Long-acting pegylated alpha-interferon (SC once a week) with oral ribavirin typically for 6 months in genotype 2/3, 12 months type 1.
- Viral response tested at 4/52 on treatment to assess likely long-term response to treatment.

Delta virus

- Blood-borne and sexually transmitted.
- 3–20 weeks incubation.
- Co-infection when HBV +ive.
- 30–50% develop chronic disease.

Hepatitis E

- Faecal-oral transmission.
- 2–9 weeks incubation.
- Endemic in India/Middle East.
- No carrier state or chronic disease.

Management

- Conservative approach is usually sufficient in acute hepatitis. Immunoglobulin treatment (5mL IM) can be considered in Hepatitis A outbreak, but is usually too late to treat contacts. Advise good hygiene. Only admit in severe attacks. Notify Public Health Officials. Patient must omit alcohol and hepatotoxic drugs. Test sexual partners of HBsAg +ive patients. If not immune give recombinant vaccine.
- **Follow-up:** recheck LFTs at 6 weeks. Advise to abstain from alcohol until LFTs recovered. Patient can resume usual activities once they feel well. This can take up to 6 weeks. If LFTs abnormal at 6 weeks recheck at 6 months, and complete full liver screen. If abnormal at 6 months liver biopsy may be warranted. Hepatitis B, C, and D can cause chronic disease.
- **Immunization:** active immunization against HAV advised if travelling to an endemic area, close contacts of patients with Hepatitis A. Passive immunization with human immunoglobulin is effective for 4 months, indicated for close contacts of patent with hepatits A (give at different site from immunoglobulin). Active immunization against hepatits B with recombinant hepatitis B vaccine – 3 doses at 0, 1, and 6 months. Indicated for HBsAg –ive contacts of HBsAg +ive patients, haemophiliacs, renal dialysis, health care personnel, workers in endemic areas. Booster every 5–10 years.
- **Hepatocellular carcinoma:** in cirrhotic patients 6 monthly USS should be performed with αFP level. Reduction in inflammation/viral load associated with reduced risk of hepatoma in hepatitis B and C. Smoking, obesity, and alcohol, increase risk and appropriate lifestyle issues should be addressed. Steroids, contraceptive pill, and HRT should be avoided.

Primary sclerosing cholangitis

- Characterized by diffuse fibrosing inflammation of intra- and extrahepatic bile ducts leading to stricturing, cholestasis, cholangitis, biliary cirrhosis, and liver failure.
- Aetiology unknown.
- Up to 90% of patients with PSC will have ulcerative colitis (UC).
- 5–10% of patients with UC will develop PSC.

Clinical features

- Asymptomatic.
- Fatigue.
- Pruritus.
- Abnormal LFTs.
- Steatorrhoea.
- Cholangitis (see Fig. 4.4).
- Gallstones.
- Obstructive jaundice.
- Cholangiocarcinoma.
- Metabolic bone disease (vitamin D deficiency).

Investigations

- LFTs. Raised ALP and GGT. ALT <300IU/L.
- IgM elevated in 30%.
- pANCA +ive in 45% (AMA usually negative).
- HLA-DRw52a +ive in 30–80%.
- **Ultrasound:** biliary dilatation if large duct stricture.
- **Cholangiography** (ERCP or MRCP): characteristic multifocal stricturing and dilatation of intra- and extrahepatic bile ducts. (**NB.** normal study in small duct PSC – pericholangitis).
- Liver biopsy may support the diagnosis, but is rarely diagnostic. Useful for staging disease.

Diagnostic criteria

- Symptoms (jaundice and pruritus).
- Persistently elevated ALP.
- Diffuse, multifocal biliary strictures (ERCP).
- Fibro-obliterative cholangitis on biopsy (rare).
- Exclude secondary causes (cholangiocarcinoma, previous biliary surgery, HIV cholangiopathy, ischaemic cholangiopathy).

Staging of PSC

- **Stage I:** enlargement/scarring of portal triad with monuclear cell infiltrate.
- **Stage II:** parenchymal fibrosis.
- **Stage III:** bridging fibrosis.
- **Stage IV:** cirrhosis.

Prognosis

- Mayo risk score (age, variceal bleeding, albumin, bilirubin, AST) superior to Child-Pugh score in predicting long-term survival.

- 10–15% lifetime risk of developing cholangiocarcinoma. Investigate dominant strictures by ERCP, brush cytology, CEA and CA19.9.

Treatment

- Ursodeoxycholic acid (15mg/kg/day) improves biochemical profile, but does not improve survival.
- Immunosuppressants and anti-inflammatory agents have no proven benefit.
- ERCP and balloon dilatation/stenting of dominant strictures.
- Colectomy for UC does not alter natural history of PSC.
- Liver transplantation: 5-year survival 85%; 20% recurrence rate.

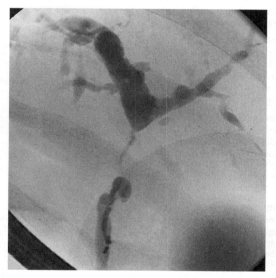

Fig. 4.4 Primary sclerosing cholangitis. Cholangiographic appearance of primary sclerosing cholangitis in a patient with a hilar stricture.

Autoimmune hepatitis

Pathology
- Aetiology of autoimmune hepatitis (AIH) unknown.
- Association with other autoimmune conditions.
- Probably initiated by a triggering event in a genetically susceptible individual (e.g. viral infection, drugs).
- HLA-DR3 +ive patients present at a younger age and have more aggressive phenotype.
- More common in women.
- Characterized by elevated autoantibody levels (e.g. ANA, ASMA, anti-LKM, AMA).
- **'Overlap syndrome':** mixed clinical and serological picture of AIH and primary biliary cirrhosis.

Clinical features
- Variable clinical presentation.
- Acute or chronic hepatitis.
- Chronic liver disease.
- Features of associated autoimmune conditions (e.g. haemolytic anaemic, ITP, eosinophilia, rheumatoid arthritis).

Investigations
- ANA (antinuclear antibody).
- ASMA (anti-smooth muscle antibody).
- Anti-LKM (anti-liver-kidney microsomal antibody).
- Serum protein electrophoresis.
- Immunoglobulin assay.
- Liver biopsy.

Diagnosis
Scoring system developed by International Autoimmune Hepatitis Group, based on multiple factors. Points scored for:
- Female sex.
- Low ALP/AST ratio.
- High IgG level.
- High autoantibody titres.
- Negative viral serology.
- Absent drug history.
- Low alcohol intake.
- Associated autoimmune disease.
- Interface hepatitis, rosetting, and/or plasma cells on biopsy.
- Response to steroid therapy.

Treatment
- Treatment is indicated if:
  - patient is symptomatic;
  - AST elevated 10-fold (or 5-fold plus gamma-globulin elevated 2-fold;
  - necrosis on biopsy.

- Start high dose oral prednisolone (initially 60mg od, tapering to 10–20mg od maintenance over 4 weeks) +/– azathioprine 50mg od.
- Treatment duration varies (up to 2 years).
- Relapse after treatment withdrawal occurs in 50% of patients and should be treated by long-term immunosuppression.
- Consider cyclosporin or tacrolimus in steroid-resistant cases.
- Patients with features of liver decompensation should be assessed for liver transplantation.
- Liver transplant associated with excellent 5-year patient (80–90%) and graft (75%) survival.
- 20–40% of patients develop recurrent AIH after transplant.
- *De novo* AIH may occur in patients transplanted for non-immune conditions.

Primary biliary cirrhosis

Pathology
- Progressive destruction of intrahepatic bile ducts, leading to cholestasis, portal inflammation, and fibrosis.
- More common in middle-aged women.

Clinical features
- Asymptomatic.
- Pruritus.
- Fatigue.
- Osteoporosis.
- Hyperlipidaemia.
- Associated autoimmune diseases.

Investigations
- Diagnostic criteria:
  - antimitochondrial antibody positivity;
  - biochemical cholestasis >6 months;
  - characteristic features on biopsy.
- Biopsy findings: cholangitis affecting interlobular bile ducts; portal inflammatory infiltrate. Fibrosis/cirrhosis in late stages.
- Consider MRCP to exclude primary sclerosing cholangitis (e.g. if AMA negative).

Prognosis
Predicted by Mayo model, based on:
- Age.
- Bilirubin.
- Albumin.
- INR.
- Severity of fluid retention.

Treatment
- Ursodeoxycholic acid (UDCA, 10–15mg/kg daily in 2–4 divided doses) is safe and improves pruritus in majority of patients. UDCA may also prevent progressive liver damage, although a survival benefit has not been clearly demonstrated.
- Cholestyramine taken before meals (4–16g daily).
- Treat associated bone disease (vitamin D and calcium supplements).
- Liver transplantation if advanced disease (e.g. intractable pruritus, complications of cirrhosis).

Non-alcoholic fatty liver disease

Definitions

Non-alcoholic fatty liver disease (NAFLD): hepatic steatosis not due to alcohol consumption. Consists of a spectrum of disorders from hepatic steatosis → non-alcoholic steatohepatitis (NASH) → fibrosis → cirrhosis.

Pathophysiology

- Common in obesity and forms part of the 'metabolic syndrome', which is characterized by hyperinsulinaemia and insulin resistance.
- Hepatic steatosis develops due to impaired mitochondrial beta-oxidation and increased hepatic lipogenesis. Progression to NASH and cirrhosis may be related to severity of metabolic syndrome.

Clinical features

- NAFLD is usually asymptomatic.
- Diagnosis may be suspected in obese patients presenting with an incidental finding of elevated ALT and AST.
- Features of chronic liver disease may be present in late stages.

Investigations

- LFTs.
- Liver biopsy.

Treatment

- Treatment of associated complications of metabolic syndrome (e.g. Diabetes, obesity, hypertension, dyslipidaemia) may prevent or slow progression of liver disease.
- Liver transplantation for patients with end-stage liver disease.

Budd-Chiari syndrome

Definition
- In 1845, George Budd, a British Physician, described 3 cases of hepatic venous thrombosis associated with abscess-induced phlebitis.
- In 1899, Hans Chiari, an Austrian pathologist, described an 'obliterating endophlebitis of the hepatic veins'.
- Thrombotic obstruction of post-sinusoidal venous outflow resulting in a congestive hepatopathy.
- Heterogenous group of disorders characterized by clinical manifestations of hepatic venous outflow occlusion at any level from the hepatic venules to the right atrium.

Epidemiology
- Worldwide prevalence 1 in 100,000.
- More common in 3rd to 4th decades.
- Women > men.

Pathogenesis
- A procoagulant disorder is identified in 75%. 25% of cases have >1 aetiological factor.
- Hepatic venous outflow can be thrombotic or non thrombotic.
- Any site from the hepatic venules to the junction of the IVC with the right atrium.
- Clinical features occur if ≥2 major hepatic veins are occluded.
- Hepatic vein occlusion → ↑ sinusoidal pressure → sinusoidal dilation → ↓ sinusoidal blood flow → venous stasis/congestion, sequestration of fluid into the interstitial space and liver congestion. In addition, portal pressure rises → ↓ portal flow → hypoxic damage to adjacent parenchyma → centrilobular hepatocyte necrosis.
- Massive hepatocellular damage → acute Budd-Chiari syndrome → acute liver failure.
- Reperfusion injury can contribute to further hepatocyte injury.
- In chronic cases, centrilobular fibrosis develops +/− nodular regenerative hyperplasia +/− cirrhosis.
- Compensatory hypertrophy of the caudate occurs in 50% of cases.
- Spontaneous porto-systemic shunt may reduce sinusoidal pressure and improve liver function.
- Portal vein thrombosis may co-exist (10–20%).

Classification
- **Primary intravascular venous thrombosis:** due to intrinsic intraluminal venous thrombosis or a vascular web/membrane.
- **Secondary:** venous thrombosis secondary to venous occlusion (e.g. extraluminal compression by tumour/cyst/abscess or intraluminal venous invasion by a tumour/parasite).

Aetiology
- Hypercoagulable states (inherited or acquired).
- Malignancy (HCC, renal, adrenal).

- Extrinsic compression (tumours, polycystic kidneys, amoebic abscess, pyogenic abscess, hydatid cyst).
- Iatrogenic (piggyback OLT, caval anastomotic stenosis, torsion of liver remnant – right lobe graft, right hepatectomy).
- Idiopathic (10%).

Hypercoagulable states

Inherited
- Protein C deficiency (25%).
- Protein S deficiency.
- Antithrombin III deficiency.
- Factor V Leiden mutation (25%). Leads to APC resistance. Associated with pregnancy and OCP.
- Prothrombin gene mutation (5%). G20210A mutation.
- Methylene tetrahydrofolate reductase gene mutation.

Acquired
- Primary myeloproliferative disorders (20% of cases). E.g. polycythaemia rubra vera, essential thrombocythaemia, myelofibrosis. A significant proportion of patients with myeloproliferative disorders have an acquired JAK2 mutation.
- Paroxysmal nocturnal haemoglobinuria (12%).
- Antiphospholipid syndrome. Anticardiolipin antibody +ive (25%).
- Hyperhomocystinemia.
- Malignancy.
- Pregnancy.
- Oral contraceptive use.
- Hormone replacement therapy.

Miscellaneous causes
- Behcet's disease (<5%).
- **Primary membranous IVC obstruction:** a sequela of IVC thrombosis without hepatic venous thrombosis (60% of cases in Asia).
- Abdominal trauma.
- Ulcerative colitis.
- Coeliac disease.
- Sarcoidosis.
- **IVC stenosis:** congenital IVC webs.

Clinical features
- Asymptomatic (5–20%).
- Abnormal LFTs.
- **Fulminant** (5%): acute liver failure, massive ascites, tender hepatomegaly, jaundice. Jaundice → encephalopathy < 8 weeks. Rapid onset of renal failure, coagulopathy, coma.
- **Acute** (20%): RUQ pain, ascites, tender hepatomegaly, jaundice. Hepatic necrosis without collateral formation. 60% have histological evidence of chronic liver disease.
- **Subacute:** onset over months. Ascites, hepatosplenomegaly +/– jaundice.
- **Chronic** (>6 months): refractory ascites with preserved liver function. Features of cirrhosis. Bilateral leg oedema suggests IVC thrombosis or compression due to caudate hypertrophy.

Investigations
- AST⇈ in fulminant BCS.
- ↑ Serum/ascitic albumin gradient.
- ↓ Protein C, protein S, and antithrombin III.
- **USS**: caudate hypertrophy, ascites, splenomegaly, HV thrombosis, or stenosis.
- **Duplex** (sensitivity/specificity >85%): absent/reduced/reversed flow in HV; intrahepatic collaterals; reduced hepatofugal flow in PV.
- Echocardiogram to exclude congestive hepatopathy.
- **Investigate for underlying cause**: blood smear; thrombophilia screen; genetic analysis for FVL and prothrombin gene mutations; bone marrow aspirate; flow cytometry for PNH; JAK2 mutation analysis.

CT appearances
- **Acute BCS:** severe ascites; hepatosplenomegaly; caudate hypertrophy; reduced peripheral enhancement; occluded HVs.
- **Chronic BCS**: ascites; peripheral liver atrophy; caudate hypertrophy; intra- and extrahepatic venous collaterals; enlarged HA; parenchymal hypoperfusion; cavernous transformation or thrombosis of PV; dilated azygos vein; regenerative nodules.

MRI appearances
- **T1-weighted images:** HV occlusion; multiple hypervascular regenerative nodules.
- **T2-weighted images**: heterogeneous hyperintensity in peripheral liver; regenerative nodules are hypointense on T2.

Liver biopsy
- Centrilobular congestion.
- Sinusoidal dilation.
- Hepatocyte necrosis.
- Cellular atrophy and fibrosis.
- Regenerative nodules.

Medical therapy
- **Indications:** partial HV occlusion; early diagnosis (days); no necrosis; contraindications to interventional treatment (comorbidity, limited life expectancy, patient refusal).
- **Anticoagulation:** IV heparin then long-term warfarin (target INR 2.5–3).
- Nutritional support.
- **Treat ascites:** low sodium diet, diuretics, paracentesis.

Interventional treatment
Thrombolysis
- Acute BCS if fresh thrombus present.
- Infuse urokinase or tPA into the thrombosed HV for 24h (transjugular or transfemoral routes).
- Most effective if performed early (<72h), but may be used up to 2–3 weeks later.

Balloon angioplasty or hepatic vein stenting
- Percutaneous or transhepatic.
- Symptomatic relief in 70%.
- High restenosis rate.
- Improved patency rates with stenting.

Laser therapy
Used for membranous IVC occlusion.

Transjugular intrahepatic portosystemic shunt
Indications: PV-infrahepatic IVC gradient <10mmHg; poor hepatic reserve; failed thromboylsis +/− angioplasty; chronic BCS; variceal bleed; bridge to liver transplantation.

Surgery
- Excise web + IVC angioplasty (if localized IVC membranous obstruction).
- **Portosystemic shunt:** if underlying cause has a favourable outcome, i.e. Child-Pugh class A; ongoing hepatic necrosis; chronic presentation without significant hepatic fibrosis; PV-infrahepatic IVC pressure gradient must be ≥10mmHg. Options include portocaval, central splenorenal, mesocaval, mesoatrial shunts.
- **Liver transplantation:** indications: fulminant BCS; end-stage liver disease; failed portosystemic shunt; inherited Protein C or S deficiency; antithrombin III deficiency.

Liver transplantation

R. Deshpande, O. Tucker, R. Sutcliffe, & P. Muiesan

General indications

- Selection of patients for transplantation is performed by a multidisciplinary team consisting of transplant surgeons, hepatologists, liver anaesthetists, liver intensivists, and transplant co-ordinators.
- In general, patients should be fit for major surgery and have a predicted 18-month survival of less than 50% if untreated, a MELD score ≥14 or UKELD score >49. Patients should have an expected post-transplant survival of at least 50% at 5 years.
- The indications for liver transplantation are listed in Table 5.1.

Timing of referral for transplant assessment

Acute liver failure
- Onset of coagulopathy.
- Onset of hepatic encephalopathy.

Chronic liver disease
- Evidence of synthetic dysfunction.
- Malnutrition (especially children).
- First major complication (variceal bleed, ascites, hepatic encephalopathy).
- Diagnosis of early HCC.

Criteria for transplant listing

Acute liver failure
- See Acute liver failure 🕮 p. 58.

Chronic liver disease
- Child-Pugh score ≥7 and/or MELD score ≥14.
- Variceal bleeding (due to portal hypertension) with decompensation.
- Recurrent encephalopathy.
- Diuretic-resistant ascites.
- Single episode of spontaneous bacterial peritonitis (SBP).
- Early hepatocellular carcinoma (within Milan criteria).

Criteria for removal from transplant list

Acute liver failure
- Active infection on high dose pressor support.
- Severe cerebral oedema with intractable intracranial hypertension.
- **NB**. One-third of patients with acute liver failure that meet transplant criteria will become untransplantable.

Chronic liver disease
- Mechanical ventilation (Hospital mortality ~95%).
- Multi-organ failure.
- MELD score >40.

Table 5.1 Indications for liver transplantation

Acute liver failure	Drug-induced hepatitis
	Paracetamol toxicity
	Acute Wilson's disease
	Acute Budd-Chiari syndrome
	Acute viral hepatitis (A, B, E)
	Seronegative hepatitis
	Primary graft non-function
	Liver trauma requiring total hepatectomy
Chronic liver disease	Viral-induced cirrhosis (hepatitis B and C)
	Alcohol-related liver disease
	Autoimmune hepatitis
	Primary biliary cirrhosis
	Secondary biliary cirrhosis
	Primary sclerosing cholangitis
	Budd-Chiari syndrome
	Cryptogenic cirrhosis
Metabolic diseases	Wilson's disease
	Haemochromatosis
	Alpha-1-antitrypsin deficiency
	Primary hyperoxaluria type 1
	Familial amyloid polyneuropathy
	Cystic fibrosis
	Progressive familial intrahepatic cholestasis (Byler's disease)
Malignancy	Hepatocellular carcinoma
	Epithelioid haemangioendothelioma
	Metastatic neuroendocrine tumour (Hepatoblastoma)
Congenital	Extrahepatic biliary atresia

Indications according to aetiology

Acute liver failure

- Transplantation should be considered in patients in whom spontaneous recovery of liver function is unlikely, e.g. acute liver failure due to hepatitis B, non-paracetamol drug-induced hepatitis, acute Wilson's disease.
- Patients with other aetiologies (e.g. acute fatty liver of pregnancy, paracetamol-induced acute liver failure, acute hepatitis A), where spontaneous recovery is possible, should be closely monitored for signs of progressive liver failure (coagulopathy, encephalopathy, acidosis) and listed accordingly.

Transplant criteria for paracetamol-induced liver failure (King's College Hospital criteria)

- pH <7.3.
- INR >6.5.
- Creatinine >300μmol/L.
- Grade III–IV hepatic encephalopathy.

Transplant criteria for non-paracetamol aetiologies of acute liver failure

- Age <10 years or >40 years.
- INR >6.5.
- Jaundice to encephalopathy time >7 days.
- Bilirubin >300μmol/L.

Chronic liver disease (Fig. 5.1)

Hepatitis B cirrhosis

- Difficult to predict natural history, usually progressive disease, but sometimes develop acute deterioration (due to viral reactivation or HBeAg seroconversion) that either improves spontaneously or progresses to acute liver failure.
- Transplant if portal hypertension (intractable ascites, SBP, variceal bleeding, encephalopathy) or liver failure.
- Post-transplant HBV re-infection develops in 80% and is predicted by pre-transplant HBV DNA status.
- Reduce risk of HBV re-infection (from 80% to 20%) by administering:
  - combination of lamivudine and adefovir, or entecovir, pre-transplant to clear HBV DNA;
  - anti-HBs immunoglobulin during anhepatic phase of transplant procedure and continue for 1 week post-transplant;
  - repeat course of anti-HBs immunoglobulin monthly in the long-term according to anti-HBs titres (aim for >100 IU/L). Give in combination with lamivudine.
  - **NB.** Studies are currently underway to determine the optimal strategy in the post-transplant setting.
- Diagnose HBV re-infection by HBsAg and HBV DNA positivity associated with progressive graft dysfunction.
- Co-infection with delta virus reduces HBV re-infection rates (delta inhibits HBV replication).

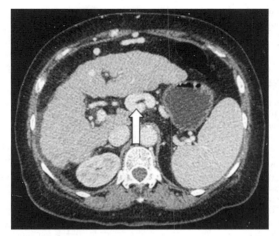

Fig. 5.1 Cirrhosis. CT appearances of macronodular cirrhosis with portal hypertension. Shrunken, heterogeneous liver, varices (arrow), splenomegaly, and ascites.

Hepatitis C cirrhosis
- 20% of patients with HCV develop cirrhosis within 20 years.
- Indications for transplant are the same as for chronic liver disease (see Indications according to aetiology, Chronic liver disease 📖 p. 92).
- Up to 30% of patients will have an associated HCC.
- 5-year post-transplant survival 75–80%.

Primary biliary cirrhosis
- Median survival in patients with PBC is 2 years when bilirubin >100µmol/L.
- Indications for transplantation are:
  - serum bilirubin >100µmol/L;
  - intractable pruritus;
  - portal hypertension;
  - hepatocellular carcinoma.
- Disease recurrence occurs in 10% at 5 years, but does not usually affect graft or patient survival.
- 10 year post-transplant survival is 80–90%.

Primary sclerosing cholangitis
- Indications for transplantation are:
  - bilirubin >100μmol/L;
  - intractable pruritus;
  - recurrent episodes of cholangitis;
  - decompensated liver disease;
  - poor quality of life.
- Prior to listing, exclude cholangiocarcinoma (30% risk at 10 years) and colorectal cancer (in IBD patients) by arranging MRCP/ERCP and colonoscopy.
- Post-transplant complications are higher in patients who have had previous interventions (e.g. biliary stents).
- 5-year post-transplant survival 73%.

Alcohol-related liver disease
- Patients can only be considered for transplantation if they have been abstinent for at least 6 months for two reasons:
  - abstinence may prevent disease progression and/or improve symptoms;
  - risk of recidivism after transplantation is high (~40%).
- Harmful drinking leading to graft loss occurs in 10–15% of patients.
- Acute alcoholic hepatitis is a contraindication to transplantation since patients are actively drinking.
- Strong psychosocial and family support are essential to maximize outcome after transplantation in this group of patients.
- Indications for transplantation are same as for chronic liver disease.

Autoimmune hepatitis/cirrhosis
- Liver biopsy is useful to assess disease activity to optimize immunosuppressive therapy (steroids/azathioprine) in order to postpone transplantation.
- Consider transplantation if decompensated cirrhosis (recurrent ascites, SBP, encephalopathy) despite optimal long-term immunosuppression.
- 5-year post-transplant survival 80%.

Budd-Chiari syndrome
- Suitability for transplantation depends on:
  - underlying cause (including status of any myeloproliferative disorders);
  - patient's clinical condition;
  - degree of hepatic vein obstruction;
  - degree of liver dysfunction.
- Consider transplantation for:
  - acute BCS with liver failure;
  - chronic BCS associated with cirrhosis unresponsive to TIPS therapy.
- Patients with prothrombotic tendencies must be anticoagulated after transplantation. Patients with JAK2 mutation are at particularly high risk of disease recurrence and must be aggressively anticoagulated. Co-existing myeloproliferative disorder should be assessed and appropriately treated.

Malignancy

Hepatocellular carcinoma

- Liver transplantation appears to be superior to resection in patients with early HCC and cirrhosis (large case-controlled series).
- Milan criteria achieve good long-term results (5-year survival 70%) and are widely used:
  - 3 or fewer tumours;
  - maximum diameter <5cm;
  - no extrahepatic disease.
- Some centres use extended criteria with similar survival (e.g. UCSF).
- Main limitation is that these criteria are based on tumour volume not biological characteristics (e.g. vascular invasion, differentation).
- Debate about the benefits of pre-transplant tumour biopsy (improved selection) vs. risks (tumour seeding).
- Fibrolamellar carcinoma. Slow growing tumours. Transplantation considered as an acceptable palliative option even for large tumours.

Cholangiocarcinoma

- Early reports of transplantation for cholangiocarcinoma were associated with high rates of recurrence.
- Excellent results (5-year survival of 71%) were reported by the Mayo clinic using neoadjuvant chemoradiotherapy in carefully selected patients. However, these results have not been widely reproduced.
- The role of liver transplantation for cholangiocarcinoma remains unproven, particularly in an era of organ shortage.

Epithelioid haemangioendothelioma

- Rare, slow growing vascular tumour, which often presents late at an unresectable stage.
- Experience of liver transplantation for this condition is limited to case reports and small series. Current role is unknown.

Neuroendocrine liver metastases

- Currently the only metastatic disease that has been accepted as an indication for liver transplantation in selected cases.
- Transplantation offers good symptomatic relief particularly for patients with carcinoid syndrome due to well-differentiated tumour.

Metabolic disorders

Cystic fibrosis

- 15% develop cirrhosis.
- Risks of transplantation increased by associated cardiopulmonary disease, malnutrition and chronic infection.

Wilson's disease

Consider liver transplantation for:
- Fulminant Wilson's with acute liver failure.
- Decompensated cirrhosis.
- Disease progression despite medical therapy
- Neurological symptoms without severe liver disease (controversial).

Alpha-1-antitrypsin deficiency
- 15% of patients with PiZZ phenotype develop liver failure by adolescence.
- Transplant if decompensated cirrhosis or liver failure.
- 5-year post-transplant survival 80%.

Hereditary tyrosinaemia
Liver transplantation should be considered early in childhood to prevent HCC (develops in a third by 2 years).

Crigler-Najjar syndrome
Transplant if phototherapy fails to improve hyperbilirubinaemia in patients with severe form (type I) of this disease.

Hereditary haemochromatosis
- Long-term venesection may prevent cirrhosis due to iron deposition.
- Transplant if decompensated cirrhosis.
- Risks of transplantation are increased due to associated cardiomyopathy and post-transplant sepsis.

Primary hyperoxaluria
- Characterized by nephrocalcinosis and renal failure.
- Treated by combined liver and renal transplantation.

Familial amyloid polyneuropathy
- Variant transthyretin produced by the liver deposits as amyloid in nerves and other organs.
- Transplantation is indicated if patient is symptomatic.
- Explanted liver may be used as a graft for another recipient (e.g. HCC patient) as a 'domino' procedure.

Paediatric disorders
- In addition to metabolic diseases, liver transplantation is also indicated for extrahepatic biliary atresia (EHBA), interlobular bile duct paucity, and Byler's disease (Progressive familial intrahepatic cholestasis, PFIC).
- If diagnosed within 3 months of birth, EHBA can be treated by Kasai portoenterostomy, which delays liver transplantation until 5–10 years of age, thereby reducing risks of transplantation.

Contraindications to liver transplantation

Technical
Portomesenteric venous thrombosis (relative contraindication).

Anaesthetic-related
- Cardiac failure.
- Respiratory failure.
- Severe pulmonary hypertension (mean PAP >55mmHg unresponsive to therapy).
- Advanced arteriopaths.

Immunosuppression-related
- Uncontrolled sepsis.
- Extrahepatic malignancy.

Compliance-related
- Ongoing drug/alcohol addiction.
- Poorly controlled psychiatric disorders.

Expanding the donor pool

- Chronic shortage of cadaveric donor organs has a significant impact on allocation of resources and patient selection.
- Transplant centres in the UK offer transplantation to potential recipients who have a predicted 5 year survival of at least 50%.
- Prolonged waiting times on the transplant list will inevitably lead to deaths before transplant.
- The cause of organ shortage is multifactorial, including ethical and religious reasons, lack of public awareness, and type of method of obtaining consent (opt-in or presumed).
- The UK operates an 'opt-in' system for organ donation. Patients may register their details on the NHS Organ Donor Register, carry a donor card, or inform their relatives of their wishes. After death, the patient's relatives are consulted for their consent before organ donation, irrespective of the patient's wishes.
- The UK Government are currently exploring the option of introducing 'presumed consent', in which patients are automatically considered as organ donors, unless they opt out. Presumed consent is practised in Spain, and has been associated with higher rates of organ donation.
- Several methods have been developed to expand the donor pool, including:
  - split liver transplantation;
  - use of marginal grafts (steatotic grafts, non-heart beating donors);
  - living related liver transplantation.
- However, these alternative approaches are not without their own disadvantages and are unlikely to lead to a significant expansion in the donor pool.
- Liver splitting is a technically demanding procedure that is only performed by few centres. Only a small proportion of heart beating cadaveric grafts are suitable (in terms of size and quality) for splitting.
- The role of living related liver transplantation remains unclear due to ongoing ethical concerns regarding donor morbidity and mortality.

Heart beating cadaveric donor hepatectomy

The organ retrieval team
- Consists of two surgeons, one scrub nurse, and one perfusionist.
- Maintains effective regular communication with the transplant centre recipient coordinator and consultant transplant surgeon.
- Shows respect for the donor and family, and staff involved in the surgery.

Pre-retrieval preparation
Check the donor medical records
- Appropriately authorized brain-death tests (Table 5.2).
- Blood group.
- Family consent.
- Age.
- Sex.
- Cause of death.
- Alcohol history.
- Smoking history.
- History of cancer (non-skin).
- Evidence of sepsis: active meningitis/bacteraemia.
- Presence of significant donor liver trauma.
- Significant pre-existing co-morbidity.
- Body mass index.
- Time in ITU (days).
- Vasopressor support.
- Episode(s) of prolonged cardiac +/– respiratory arrest.
- Urea and electrolyte levels particularly serum sodium.
- Liver function tests.
- HBsAg, HBcAb, and HCV Ab status.
- HTLV-1 and -2, HIV serology.
- Establish identity of the donor: check the patient's name tag with details in the medical records.

Establish an effective collaborative relationship
With:
- Local donor co-ordinator.
- Local anaesthetist.
- Local theatre staff.
- Local porters.
- Other retrieval teams (cardiothoracic, renal, etc.)

Surgical techniques
- Standard retrieval.
- Rapid retrieval.
- *En bloc* retrieval.

Table 5.2 Brain stem death criteria.

Preconditions	There should be no doubt that the patient's condition is due to IRREMEDIABLE brain damage of known aetiology
	The patient is deeply unconscious
	The following conditions are excluded: drug intoxication, hypothermia, metabolic or endocrine disturbance, cardiovascular instability
Tests	
1	Pupils are fixed and dilated
2	Absent corneal reflex
3	Absent vestibulo-ocular reflexes
4	Absent motor response within cranial nerve distribution
5	Absent gag reflex
6	Absent respiratory movements (disconnect ventilator and allow $PaCO_2$ to rise >6.65kPa)

The diagnosis of brain stem death should be made by at least two doctors >5 years post-registration (one must be a consultant and neither can be members of the transplant team). The tests can be carried out separately or together. The legal time of death is when the first set of tests has indicated brain stem death.

Standard retrieval technique

Preparation and access
- Standard sterilization and draping of the patient.
- Laparotomy and median sternotomy.
  - full length midline incision from suprasternal notch to pubic symphysis;
  - open abdominal cavity;
  - divide sternum in the midline and apply bone wax to the bony edges;
  - position thoracic and abdominal retractors.
- Open pericardium.
- Place moist small swab over heart.
- Divide round ligament.
- Inspect liver and other intra-abdominal organs.

Warm dissection phase
- **Liver mobilization:**
  - divide falciform and left triangular ligaments;
  - divide adhesions around the liver and gallbladder;
  - check for accessory left hepatic artery (LHA) arising from the left gastric artery;
  - inspect gastro-hepatic ligament for an accessory LHA;
  - completely divide the ligament if accessory LHA absent;
  - if present, partially divide the ligament with preservation of the artery.
- Check for accessory RHA arising from the superior mesenteric artery or coeliac trunk, by palpating for pulsation in the right side of porta hepatis.
- Do not mobilize right lobe.

- **Porta hepatis dissection:**
  - divide small superficial veins and right gastric artery close to the duodenum;
  - ligate and divide the gastroduodenal artery leaving a reasonable stump – before division ensure the gastroduodenal artery is not the main arterial supply to the liver. If in doubt preserve it;
  - identify, ligate, and divide the distal common bile duct (CBD);
  - identify and encircle the splenic artery on the superior aspect of the pancreas – do not ligate or divide the splenic artery;
  - ensure there is no misidentification of the common hepatic artery for the splenic artery;
  - avoid the use of traction, which may cause arterial intimal injury (see Fig. 5.2).
- **Infrahepatic vena cava dissection:**
  - mobilize the second part of the duodenum using the kocher manoeuvre;
  - identify the IVC and the renal veins (the right renal vein lies lower than the left);
  - encircle the IVC above the level of the renal veins;
  - place a vessel loop around the encircled IVC and secure with a small artery clip.

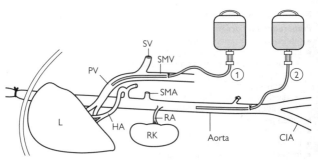

Fig. 5.2. Aortic and portal cannulation. 1: Portal vein cannula, 2: Aortic cannula, L: liver, RK: right kidney, PV: portal vein, SV: splenic vein, SMV: superior mesenteric vein, HA: hepatic artery, RA: renal artery, SMA: superior mesenteric artery, CIA: common iliac artery.

- **Aortic dissection:**
  - mobilize the small bowel so that the loops can be displaced to the patient's left upper quadrant;
  - identify the lower end of the abdominal aorta between the origin of the inferior mesenteric artery and origin of the common iliac arteries at the bifurcation;
  - expose and encircle the lower aorta with two heavy vicryl ties or a nylon tape if atheromatous; if significant atheroma, dissect and encircle both common iliac arteries for cannulation.

- **Superior mesenteric vein dissection:**
  - the first assistant lifts the transverse colon upwards to expose the root of the small bowel mesentery;
  - commence the mesenteric dissection 3cm inferior to the insertion of the mesocolon;
  - with careful dissection identify the SMV;
  - ligate and divide any tributaries;
  - encircle the SMV with 2 heavy vicryl ties and secure with a small artery clip.
- **Supra-coeliac aorta dissection:**
  - with the assistant gently retracting the liver laterally, identify the supra-coeliac space posterior to the left lateral segment of the liver;
  - separate the crural fibres, avoiding the oesophagus and identify the infra-diaphragmatic aorta;
  - isolate the aorta with a Semb clamp and encircle with a nylon tape;
  - in the presence of an accessory LHA, isolate and encircle the supra-diaphragmatic aorta through the chest

Cannulation
- The perfusionist prepares the perfusate and catheters.
- Adequate perfusate flow through both catheters (for dual perfusion) is checked by the surgeon.
- Ensure an absence of bubbles in the cannulation system.
- Prior to cannulation ask the anesthetist to administer intravenous heparin:
  - *adult* – 20,000U heparin in a standard 70kg male;
  - *children* – 400 IU/kg.
- **Aortic cannulation:**
  - the assistant retracts the proximal lower aortic tie upwards;
  - the lower vicryl tie is ligated occluding the distal aorta near the bifurcation;
  - the surgeon compresses the proximal aorta against the vertebral column with the left hand, while making a horizontal incision in the anterior aortic wall;
  - an atheromatous-free area of the aorta should be selected;
  - introduce and advance the aortic catheter;
  - position the catheter below the level of the renal arteries;
  - ensure adequate back flow of blood to check intraluminal position;
  - the assistant secures the catheter by ligating the proximal tie;
  - an arterial clip is placed below the catheter entry site to provide further aortic occlusion.
- **Portal cannulation:**
  - the assistant retracts the proximal SMV tie upwards.
  - ligate the lower vicryl tie to occlude the proximal SMV.
  - create a horizontal anterior SMV venotomy.
  - introduce the cannula;
  - ensure adequate back flow of blood to check intraluminal position;
  - position the catheter in the proximal portal vein
  - if the catheter position is too high, unilateral liver perfusion will occur, while if the catheter position is too low, migration into the splenic vein with lack of portal perfusion will occur;

- the assistant secures the catheter by ligation of the proximal tie;
- if the pancreas is also being retrieved, cannulate the portal vein directly above the pancreas and divide the portal vein proximal to the cannula.

Exsanguination
- Agree the timing of aortic cross-clamping with other retrieval teams, anaesthetist, scrub nurse, and perfusionist.
- Have two suction devices ready and working.
- Divide the supra-diaphragmatic IVC, maintaining sufficient length to facilitate the recipient caval anastomosis.
- Dual perfusion:
  - commence aortic perfusion (3L Marshall's solution);
  - commence portal perfusion (1L University of Wisconsin solution);
  - clamp the supra-coeliac aorta;
  - ensure adequate perfusate flow;
  - ensure adequate liver perfusion;
  - assess degree of fatty infiltration.

Perfusate solution for organ retrieval

- **Adults** (liver/kidney):
  - 3L Marshall's solution for aortic perfusion;
  - 1L University of Wisconsin solution (UW) for portal perfusion.
- **Adults** (pancreas): 1L of UW solution for aortic perfusion.
- **Children** (<40kg body weight): UW solution for both aortic and portal perfusion.

Gallbladder and biliary tree flush
- Open the gallbladder fundus.
- Aspirate gallbladder contents.
- Flush the gallbladder with cold saline using a syringe.
- Open proximal end of CBD.
- Remove CBD ligature and flush CBD with cold saline *until clear*.

Hepatectomy
- Divide the diaphragm perpendicular to the hepatic veins.
- Mobilize the right lobe of the liver.
- Divide the encircled infrahepatic IVC.
- After 1L portal perfusate instilled, remove the catheter, divide and mobilize the portal vein.
- Divide the distal SMA. Preserve accessory RHA if present.
- Divide the encircled splenic artery.
- Preserve accessory LHA if present by dissection on the lesser gastric curvature.
- Continue dissection from coeliac trunk to aorta.
- Stop aortic perfusion after 3L, and divide the supra-coeliac aorta.
- Identify the SMA origin.
- Cut an aortic patch to include the SMA origin in the presence of an accessory RHA.
- Remove the liver.

Liver perfusion on the bench
- Ensure no bubbles present in the cannulation system.
- Perform hepatic arterial (600mL) and portal (600mL) perfusion with UW solution.
- Assess liver graft characteristics:
  - capsular tears/haematoma;
  - liver mass;
  - consistency;
  - degree of fat infiltration;
  - adequacy of perfusion.
- Flush the CBD with 200mL UW solution.

Packing
- Maintain sterility.
- Place the liver in a sterile bowl and completely cover with UW solution at 4°C.
- Enclose the liver in a series of three sterile plastic bags.
- Remove air from the bowl.
- Put cold saline & ice slush between the second and third bags.
- Place the liver in an ice-box.

Interaction with other retrieval teams
- Be helpful and polite.
- Allow the other surgeons to inspect the heart/lungs/pancreas/kidneys.
- Maintain good communication.
- To optimize multi-organ retrieval establish a common agreement and management plan in relation to:
  - cannulation: single or dual perfusion?
  - timing of aortic cross-clamping;
  - supra-diaphragmatic IVC clamping;
  - the length of the supra-diaphragmatic IVC (cardiothoracic team);
  - the length of the infra-diaphragmatic IVC (renal team);
  - perfusion pressure, flow, and volume.

Other tissues to be retrieved
- Bilateral iliac arteries.
- Bilateral iliac veins.
- SMA (optional for split liver transplantation).
- Spleen for tissue typing (minimum 5 samples).
- Lymph nodes for cross-matching (minimum 10).

Completion of the procedure
- Aspirate fluid/blood from the thorax and abdomen.
- Close the skin with continuous nylon suture.
- Complete the donor retrieval documentation.
- Write a brief operative note in the patient's medical records.
- Communicate with the liver transplant consultant on call.
- Last offices.

Alternative retrieval techniques
Rapid retrieval
- Multiorgan retrieval.

- A means of rapid procurement of all abdominal organs.
- Initially used in hemodynamic ally unstable donors.
- Subsequently used by some centres for all multiorgan retrievals.

Technique
- Standard sterilization and draping of the patient.
- Laparotomy and thoracotomy.
- '*In situ*' flush:
  - immediate cannulation of aorta and SMV;
  - establish cold perfusion.
- Cold dissection technique.
- Use meticulous dissection to avoid damaging vital structures.
- Reported advantages over standard retrieval technique:
  - simplification of the procedure enables less experienced surgeons to perform successful organ retrieval;
  - lower incidence of organ damage during retrieval.

En-bloc retrieval
- ≥2 Abdominal organs are removed together from the donor.
- Separation of the organs is performed by dissection on the back table at ice temperature.
- Liver, pancreas, and kidneys can be retrieved in 1.5–2.25h.
- Reported advantages:
  - shorter retrieval times;
  - shorter mean dissection time;
  - reduced primary graft non-function rates;
  - less organ damage during retrieval;
  - reduced episodes of acute pancreatitis with improved early function in pancreas grafts with *en bloc* liver and pancreas retrieval;
  - improved liver function and shorter mean hospital stay with *en bloc* liver and pancreas retrieval.
- Rapid *en bloc* technique with *in situ* aortic cooling can be used in unstable donors.

Non-heart beating cadaveric donor hepatectomy

Definitions
- **Non-heart beating donor** (NHBD): a donor whose death is defined by irreversible cessation of circulatory and respiratory functions.
- **There are two categories of NHBD:**
  - *Controlled* – donor death occurs within an intensive care unit/hospital with planned treatment withdrawal by a consultant physician/intensivist/neurosurgeon. The decision to withdraw life support should be in the patient's best interest after discussion with the family and independent of any consideration of donor suitability.
  - *Uncontrolled* – donors who suffer unexpected cardiorespiratory arrest outside or within the hospital, where resuscitation attempts have failed to restore cardiac function. The organs are retrieved after a standoff period during which death is certified.
- NHBDs are further categorized into 4 groups by location and mode of death according to the Maastricht classification (see Table 5.3).
  - *categories I, II, IV* – uncontrolled donor;
  - *categories III, IV* – controlled donor.
- Stand-off period. Period between asystole and organ retrieval:
  - University of Pittsburgh Medical Center, USA 2min;
  - the Institute of Medicine, USA 5min;
  - British Transplantation Society and Intensive Care Society 5min;
  - Maastricht Statements and Recommendations 10min.

Ethical issues
- **Controlled donation:**
  - cultural perspective of death;
  - use of premortem procedures or medications to improve organ preservation;
  - standardization of protocols on stand-off time between cardiac arrest and organ retrieval.
- **Uncontrolled donation:**
  - obtaining prompt family consent;
  - non-consensual preservation methods to facilitate option for donation until consent available;
  - protocol standardization on methods and duration of resuscitation attempts;
  - determination and declaration of death;
  - timing of death;
  - timing of organ retrieval;
  - recipient's consent;
  - implied consent (Spain).

Table 5.3 Maastricht classification of non-heart beating donors (1995)

Stage	Classification
I	Declared dead at a non-hospital site
II	Unsuccessful resuscitation attempt
III	Ventilatory support is removed from hospitalized patients with irreversible brain damage insufficient to declare brain death and cardiac death awaited
IV	Brain stem death is declared before unanticipated or anticipated cardiac arrest

Uncontrolled liver donation
- When a potential category I or II donor suffers a cardiac arrest, and all attempts at CPR have failed, CPR is suspended for a stand-off period of 5min.
- The donor is declared dead.
- CPR is resumed.
- Consent for donation is sought from the patient's family.
- The retrieval team is contacted.
- The femoral vessels are cannulated.
- Organ preservation can be achieved by two methods:
  - cardiopulmonary support (CPS) with simultaneous application of chest and abdominal compression;
  - hypothermic or normothermic cardiopulmonary bypass establishing an extracorporeal membrane oxygenation (ECMO) circuit until cold preservation is established at retrieval.
- Once consent has been obtained the retrieval process commences.

Retrieval process
- **Phase 1:** dissection phase while on ECMO.
- **Phase 2**: cardiopulmonary support/ECMO discontinued.
- **Phase 3**: organ perfusion with cold preservation solution with retrieval using standard technique.

Controlled liver donation
- The retrieval team arrives at the donating hospital before the withdrawal procedure is commenced.
- The death is certified by a consultant physician following asystole with a stand-off period of 5min.
- The patient is rapidly transferred into the operating theatre.

Surgical technique
Modifications of super-rapid technique described by Casavilla et al (1995).

Preparation and access
Standard sterilization and draping of the patient.

Standard retrieval technique
- Midline laparotomy. Full length midline incision from suprasternal notch to pubic symphysis.
- Median sternotomy.

- Divide the IVC at the level of the right atrium and drain to ease intra-abdominal organ congestion due to cardiac failure and arrest.
- Position thoracic and abdominal retractors.
- Rapidly isolate and cannulate the distal aorta with a large bore (size no. 20) cannula followed by perfusion with fibrinolytic agent (streptokinase/rTPA) and cold Marshall 's solution containing 20,000U of heparin.
- Clamp the descending aorta above the diaphragm with a large clamp to direct the perfusate towards the splanchnic organs.

Cold dissection technique
- Cannulate the superior mesenteric vein and position the catheter in the proximal portal vein.
- Perfuse the liver with cold University of Wisconsin solution containing 20,000U of heparin.
- Cool the abdominal cavity with saline ice slush.
- Open the gallbladder fundus and aspirate the contents.
- Divide the common bile duct.
- Flush the gallbladder and CBD with abundant cold saline until clear.
- Open the lesser sac.
- Divide the gastroduodenal artery, splenic, and left gastric arteries.
- Remove the portal cannula after perfusion of 1L of UW solution and divide the portal vein at the junction with the splenic vein or shorter if pancreatic retrieval planned.
- Retrieve an aortic patch with the SMA origin in the presence of an accessory RHA.
- Divide the IVC just above the origin of the renal veins.
- Extra care should be taken to avoid damage to an accessory or replaced left or right hepatic artery due to absence of pulsation to aid identification in the cold dissection phase.

Hepatectomy
- Divide the diaphragm perpendicular to the hepatic veins.
- Mobilize the right lobe of the liver.
- Divide the encircled infrahepatic IVC.
- Preserve accessory LHA if present by dissection on the lesser gastric curvature.
- Remove the liver.
- The remainder of the procedure is identical to heart-beating cadaveric donor hepatectomy (see Heart-beating cadaveric donor hepatectomy 📖 p. 105).

Further information

Casavilla, A., Ramirez, C., Shapiro, R., Nghiem, D., Miracle, K., Bronsther, O., Randhawa, P., Broznick, B., Fung, J.J., Starzl, T. (1995) Experience with liver and kidney allografts from non-heart-beating donors. *Transplantation*, **59**, 197–203

Orthotopic liver transplantation

Intraoperative monitoring and access
- Invasive BP, CVP monitoring.
- Urinary catheter.
- Consider CO monitoring (e.g. Swan-Ganz catheter or PiCCO).
- Large bore right internal jugular vein rapid infuser.
- Thromboelastography.

Incision
Mercedes.

Recipient hepatectomy
- Mobilize both lobes of the liver as described in 'left hepatectomy' and 'right hepatectomy'.
- Dissect the hilum and divide the CBD, common hepatic artery, and portal vein.
- Divide the IVC above and below the liver.
- Excise the native liver.

Implantation
- Donor IVC-recipient IVC end-to-end anastomosis (4/0 prolene). An alternative is the 'piggyback' implantation – end-to-side anastomosis (see Fig. 5.3).
- Flush liver with saline via portal vein to clear preservation fluid (containing potassium).
- Donor portal vein-recipient portal vein end-to-end anastomosis (6/0 prolene).
- Donor hepatic artery-recipient hepatic artery (6/0 or 7/0 prolene).
- Reconstruct donor right accessory artery using donor iliac artery graft as a conduit (pass through window in transverse mesocolon and anastomose to infracolic aorta).
- Remove clamps on IVC, hepatic artery and portal vein to reperfuse the liver. Inform the anaesthetist before reperfusing (risk of significant cardiovascular instability +/– cardiac arrest).
- Ensure perfect haemostasis at vascular anastomoses.

Biliary anastomosis
- Cleanly divide donor bile duct about 1cm below the hilar confluence.
- Perform an end-to-end anastomosis between donor and recipient bile ducts using 5/0 or 6/0 PDS interrupted sutures.
- Insert a T-tube if there is a size discrepancy between donor and recipient ducts.
- Reconstruct with a 50cm retrocolic Roux-en-Y hepaticojejunostomy in selected cases:
  - diseased recipient bile duct (e.g. PSC);
  - inadequate donor bile duct length (e.g. right lobe graft);
  - gross size mismatch;
  - re-transplantation.

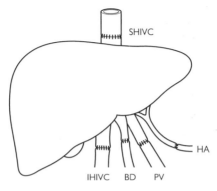

(a) **Standard technique – Anastomoses**

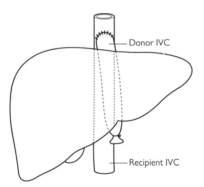

(b) **Piggyback technique**

Fig. 5.3 Orthotopic liver transplant. (a) Standard technique. Anastomoses.
(b) Piggyback technique. SHIVC: suprahepatic inferior vena cava, IHIVC: infrahepatic
inferior vena cava, BD: bile duct, PV: portal vein, HA: hepatic artery.

Split liver transplantation

- A whole liver can be split in two and implanted into two recipients:
  - left lateral segment (paediatric recipient) and extended right lobe (adult recipient; see Fig. 5.4); the graft is divided to the right of the falciform ligament;
  - left and right lobes (two adult recipients) – the graft is divided along the principal plane; the middle hepatic vein may be kept on one half, or transected and reconstructed using donor iliac vein ('MHV split' technique, see Fig. 5.4).
- Splitting of a donor liver may be performed *in situ* or *ex situ*, each with their own potential advantages. Both approaches yield comparable patient and graft outcomes in experienced hands.
- Both techniques require in depth knowledge of the anatomy of the liver segments, bile ducts, hepatic arteries, and portal veins, including an awareness of anatomical anomalies.

In situ split

- The donor liver is transected in the warm dissection phase of the retrieval procedure.
- This allows two grafts to be used by different centres without prolonged cold ischaemic times.
- This method allows accurate and meticulous haemostasis at the cut surface, to reduce bleeding in the recipient after implantation.
- However, this procedure adds significant time and complexity to the retrieval operation.
- Relies on additional resources provided by the donor hospital (e.g. CUSA and argon).

Ex situ split

- The donor liver is transected on the back table at the recipient centre, using the 'crush clamp' technique.
- Vessels and ducts on the cut surfaces are carefully ligated and divided.
- Increased risk of cut surface bleeding after implantation compared to *in situ* splitting.
- Risk of inadvertent warming during splitting, leading to warm ischaemic injury.

Reduced liver transplantation

- Similar in principle to split liver transplantation, except only one part of the liver graft is used for transplantation. Technique of reduction was developed before splitting.
- **Indication:** to improve size matching between liver graft and intended recipient (in terms of graft-body weight ratio).
- A whole liver can be reduced in three ways to provide grafts based on the segmental anatomy of the liver.
- **Left lateral segment graft.**
  - segments II and III;
  - enables donor to recipient size reduction of 10:1;
  - the recipient's native liver is excised with preservation of the IVC;

- the donor graft is piggybacked onto the recipient's IVC by anastomosing the left hepatic vein to the common orifice of the hepatic veins with a triangulation technique to reduce the risk of outflow obstruction.
- **Left lobe graft:**
  - segments II–IV;
  - enables donor to recipient size reduction of 3:1.
- **Right lobe graft:**
  - segments V–VIII;
  - enables donor to recipient size reduction of 1.5:1.

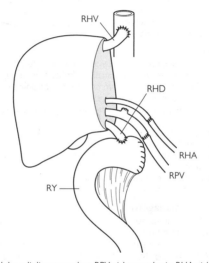

Fig. 5.4 Right lobe split liver transplant. RPV: right portal vein, RHA: right hepatic artery, RHD: right hepatic duct, RHV: right hepatic vein, RY: Roux-en-Y hepatico-jejunostomy.

Auxiliary liver transplantation

Principle
- Implantation of a reduced graft with part of the native liver left *in situ* (see Fig. 5.5).
- Selective use in patients less than 40 years old with acute liver failure (e.g. paracetamol-induced) in whom native liver expected to regenerate (e.g. no fibrosis on biopsy).
- Transplanted liver temporarily replaces liver function to allow patient to recover.
- After native liver regeneration, immunosuppression is withdrawn to allow the transplanted liver to be rejected and atrophy.
- Prevents long-term sequelae of immunosuppression (e.g. malignancy) in otherwise fit, young patients.

Technique
- Patient must be haemodynamically and neurologically stable.
- Partial recipient hepatectomy (usually right hepatectomy) is performed to allow sufficient space to accommodate the transplanted liver.
- Reduced (or split) right lobe is engrafted:
  - donor right hepatic artery anastomosed to recipient aorta via iliac conduit;
  - donor right portal vein anastomosed end-to-end to recipient right portal vein stump;
  - donor IVC anastomosed end-to-side to recipient IVC (piggyback technique);
  - donor right hepatic duct reconstructed using Roux-en-Y hepatico-jejunostomy.

Postoperative management
- Recovery from multi-organ failure and intracranial hypertension is prolonged compared with standard orthotopic liver transplant for acute liver failure, since part of the necrotic native liver is left *in situ*.
- Graft dysfunction may be difficult to evaluate. Low threshold for biopsying the transplanted liver.
- Repeat CT scans in the follow-up period to assess volume of native liver and confirm adequate regeneration prior to withdrawing immunosuppression.

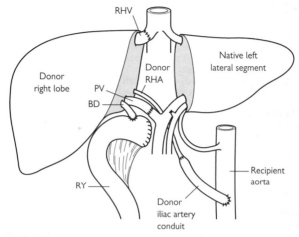

Fig. 5.5 Auxiliary liver transplant. RHV: right hepatic vein, PV: portal vein, BD: donor bile duct, RY: Roux-en-Y hepatico-jejunostomy.

Living donor hepatectomy

- The procedure involves removing a portion of normal liver from a healthy living donor for transplantation into a recipient with end-stage liver disease.
- The weight of liver tissue to be transplanted should be approximately 0.8% of the recipient's body weight.
- Paediatric recipients usually receive a left lateral segment graft and adult recipients receive a right lobe graft.

Preoperative donor assessment

- Evaluate donor for presence of cardiorespiratory comorbidity and optimize as far as possible. Evaluate for prothrombotic tendencies (e.g. procoagulant screen), smoking history and use of contraceptive pill.
- Evaluate the donor's hepatic anatomy (i.e. identify arterial and biliary anomalies) to minimize risk of intraoperative injury. Preoperative CT with 3-D reconstruction of vascular and biliary structures.

Living donor right hepatectomy

- Donor hepatectomy is similar in principle to standard liver resection, but with some important differences, based on the principles that the portion of liver to be resected must remain viable, and have a bile duct, hepatic artery, and portal and hepatic vein branches suitable for anastomosis.
- Inflow and outflow is maintained during parenchymal transection.
- Detailed evaluation of the anatomy of the donor segment is required, including intraoperative cholangiography.
- Incision as per standard right hepatectomy (Mercedes or J-shaped).
- Perform a cholecystectomy and cholangiography via the cystic duct stump.
- Perform intraoperative ultrasound to map the position of the middle hepatic vein, and determine whether segments 5 and/or 8 drain into it.
- Identify and encircle the right hepatic artery avoiding excessive dissection (to prevent ischaemic injury to the bile duct).
- Identify and dissect the portal venous bifurcation.
- Mobilize the liver off the IVC and encircle the right hepatic vein.
- Parenchymal transection is performed (see Right hepatectomy 📖).
- Divide the right hepatic duct flush with the parenchyma, and ligate the donor side.
- Cleanly divide the inflow and outflow vessels after clamping the donor side.
- Perfuse the resected liver immediately with cold UW solution.
- Ligate cut surface leaks with 4/0 prolene sutures.
- Ligate the divided donor vessels as per standard hepatectomy.

Anatomical variations

- **Accessory right hepatic artery:**
  - clearly identify and dissect;
  - if it is a true accessory artery (main right hepatic artery is also present), preserve both arteries and graft to the recipient hepatic artery using one or two anastomoses.

- Insertion of right anterior and/or posterior sectoral duct into left main hepatic duct:
  - the aberrant duct must be clearly identified and divided flush with parenchyma;
  - anastomose to the recipient bile duct separate to the main donor hepatic duct.
- **Accessory hepatic veins:**
  - preserve large inferior hepatic veins (>0.5cm) and implant directly onto the recipient IVC;
  - tributaries from segments V and VIII to the middle hepatic vein should also be separately implanted onto the recipient IVC to prevent congestion.

Living donor left lateral segmentectomy

- Dissect the hilum to expose the left hepatic artery and left portal vein.
- The segment IV artery from the left hepatic artery may be divided to gain adequate length for implantation.
- An accessory left hepatic artery must be dealt with in a similar way as described for right donor hepatectomy.
- Branches of the portal vein to segment I are also divided.
- Parenchymal transection is performed.
- Divide the left hepatic duct flush with the parenchymal surface.
- Clearly identify anomalies in biliary anatomy, and deal with to prevent postoperative bile leak. Continuous suture of the portal plate to oversew caudate biliary radicles.
- After hepatotomy, divide the inflow and outflow and cold-perfuse the resected segment on the back table.

Complications after living donor hepatectomy

Donor complications
- See Right hepatectomy 📖 p. 184.
- Cut surface leaks (2–5%).
- Bleeding (transfusion requirement in 2%).
- Donor mortality is very rare (0.2–0.5%), but is a major factor that limits more widespread use of living donor liver transplantation. Donor mortality after left lateral segment donation is approximately 1 in 1500.
- Incisional hernia 10%.

Recipient complications
See Split liver transplantation 📖 p. 114.

Living related liver transplantation

- Excision of the left lateral segment from a parent donor with transplantation into a child.
- Implantation using the piggyback technique.
- 1-year graft survival >90%.
- 1-year patient survival 95%.
- Living donor liver transplant is an option for the majority of patients, but should be reserved as a second-line choice if cadaveric split donor grafts are available.

Advantages over cadaveric transplantation

- Planned elective procedure.
- Avoids prolonged waiting list time.
- Extensive preoperative donor assessment is performed to ensure suitability and a compatible size match for the recipient.
- Blood group match.
- Excellent early graft function.
- Shorter overall hospital stay.

Disadvantages

- No short-term immunological advantage over cadaveric grafts.
- Donor mortality rate.
- Donor morbidity rate 5%: bile leak, haemorrhage, risk of splenectomy, postoperative small bowel obstruction, incisional hernia.

Complications

- Primary non-function. Less than 1% of patients.
- **Vascular:**
  - hepatic artery thrombosis;
  - portal vein thrombosis.
- **Caval obstruction:** suprahepatic caval stenosis.
- **Biliary:**
  - bile leaks;
  - biliary strictures (anastomotic or non-anastomotic).
- **Roux loop hepatico-jejunostomy-related:**
  - bile leak;
  - stricture.
- Bowel perforation.
- Infection.
- Toxicity of immunosuppressive drugs.
- Renal insufficiency/nephrotoxicity.
- Hypertension.
- *De novo* autoimmune hepatitis.
- Chronic rejection.
- Malignancy.
- Lymphoproliferative disorders.
- Delayed cholecystectomy.
- Mortality.

Paediatric liver transplantation

Indications
- **Acute liver failure:**
  - viral or drug-induced;
  - fatty acid oxidation defects;
  - neonatal haemochromatosis;
  - tyrosinaemia type 1;
  - acute Wilson's disease;
- **Chronic liver disease:**
  - biliary atresia;
  - progressive familial intrahepatic cholestasis (PFIC, Byler's disease);
  - Alagille syndrome;
  - idiopathic neonatal hepatitis;
  - alpha-1-antitrypsin deficiency;
  - Wilson's disease;
  - cystic fibrosis;
  - glycogen storage disease types I and IV;
  - total parenteral nutrition-induced cholestasis;
  - autoimmune hepatitis;
  - sclerosing cholangitis;
  - hepatitis B/C cirrhosis;
  - fibropolycystic liver disease;
  - Budd-Chiari syndrome;
  - cryptogenic cirrhosis;
  - tyrosinaemia type 1.
- **Inborn errors of metabolism:**
  - Crigler-Najjar syndrome type 1;
  - familial hypercholesterolaemia;
  - organic acidaemia;
  - urea cycle defects;
  - primary hyperoxaluria.
- **Unresectable liver tumours:**
  - haemangioendothelioma;
  - hepatoblastoma.

Prerequisites for successful paediatric liver transplantation
- Donor and recipient should be ABO blood group compatible, but preferably ABO matched.
- Donor age ≤50 years.
- Satisfactory donor liver function.
- Negative donor virology for hepatitis A, B, C, and HIV.
- Appropriate size-match or surgically size reduced graft.

Types of graft used
- **Cadaveric liver transplantation:**
  - whole graft;
  - split graft;
  - reduced graft.

- **Living related liver transplantation:**
  - left lateral lobe;
  - left lobe;
  - right lobe.

Survival

One-year survival after liver transplantation for chronic liver disease is 80–90%.

Post-transplant management

General
- Elective ITU admission for 24h.
- Early extubation if uncomplicated procedure, no significant post-reperfusion syndrome, patient stable, and good graft function.
- Continuation of organ support and intracranial pressure monitoring until recovery in patients with acute liver failure.
- Epidural analgesia usually contraindicated due to coagulopathy.
- Allow sips of water po initially. Gradually build up oral intake (fluid followed by diet) as tolerated over 2–3 days. If Roux-en-Y hepaticojejunostomy, allow only sips of water until day 3.
- Daily review by transplant hepatologist and transplant surgeon.
- Daily blood tests (FBC, U&E, LFTs, INR).
- Routine duplex US to exclude hepatic artery or portal vein thrombosis on days 1 and 5.
- Thromboprophylaxis (TED stockings and sc LMW heparin) unless coagulopathy. Restart therapeutic anticoagulation in patients with Budd-Chiari syndrome due to prothrombotic disorder.
- Give Valganciclovir (IV followed by oral) for 3 months post-transplant to prevent cytomegalovirus-related complications in high risk cases (donor CMV IgG positive, recipient negative), where the risk of CMV disease is >70%. Alternatively, selective policy of monitoring CMV PCR status, treating patients if positive.

Immunosuppression
See Table 5.4 for details of immunosuppressive drugs used in liver transplantation.
- Regimen used depends on unit protocol (e.g. tacrolimus and reducing dose of prednisolone).
- Monitoring of therapeutic levels advised for tacrolimus, cyclosporine, sirolimus, and mycophenolate mofetil.
- It is possible to reduce the immunosuppressant dose after several months or years, provided that graft function is normal.
- Tacrolimus monotherapy may be sufficient in the long-term.
- Patients with immune-based liver disease should be maintained on low dose prednisolone, as well as tacrolimus.
- Immunosuppressant dose should also be reduced or switched if evidence of significant renal impairment. Add mycophenolate mofetil to allow reduced dose of tacrolimus. Add sirolimus to allow withdrawal of tacrolimus.
- High dose 'pulsed' methyprednisolone (1g/day for 3 days) is used to treat severe acute cellular rejection. Second-line options include rabbit antithymocyte globulin (ATG) or IL-2 receptor antagonists (e.g. Dacluzimab).

Table 5.4 Immunosuppressive drugs used in liver transplantation

Drug	Mechanisms of action	Side effects
Corticosteroids, e.g. prednisolone	Inhibit macrophages Inhibit arachidonic acid metabolism Inhibit MHC Class II expression	Infections, myopathy, diabetes, bruising, centripetal obesity, abdominal striae, psychosis, poor wound healing, pancreatitis
Azathioprine	Inhibits lymphocyte proliferation	Infections, bone marrow suppression, pancreatitis, malignancy
Cyclosporin A (Neoral)	Binds cyclophilin and inhibits calcineurin leading to inhibition of IL-2 transcription	Renal failure, gum hyperplasia, seizures, hirsutism, peptic ulcers, pancreatitis, confusion, paraesthesia, infections, malignancy
Tacrolimus (Prograf, Advagraf)	Binds FKBP and inhibits calcineurin leading to inhibition of IL-2 transcription	Renal failure, hypertension, diabetes, neuropathy, seizures, infections, malignancy
Rapamycin (Sirolimus)	Binds FKBP and inhibits mTOR pathway	Poor wound healing, hyperlipidaemia, infection, malignancy, hypertension
Mycophenolate mofetil (MMF)	Inhibits inosine monophosphate dehydrogenas, blocking the purine synthesis pathway	Nausea/vomiting, diarrhoea, leukopaenia, anaemia, teratogenesis, skin rash, hypertension, infections, malignancy, progressive multifocal leukoencephalopathy
Rabbit antithymocyte globulin	Induce complement-mediated lysis of lymphocytes	Fever, nausea, arrhythmias, anaphylaxis
Dacluzimab (Zenapax)	Humanized anti-IL-2 receptor antagonist	Hypersensitivity reactions (rare)

Graft dysfunction

Causes

Preservation injury
Primary non-function.

Rejection
- Hyperacute.
- Acute.
- Chronic.

Technical complications
- Hepatic artery thrombosis.
- Portal vein stenosis or thrombosis.
- Venous outflow obstruction.
- Bile leak.
- Biliary stricture.

Infection
- Bacterial.
- Viral.
- Fungal.

Disease recurrence
- Hepatitis C.
- Alcohol recidivism.
- Hepatitis B.
- Primary biliary cirrhosis.
- Primary sclerosing cholangitis.
- Autoimmune hepatitis.
- Budd-Chiari syndrome.

General approach

- Clinical and biochemical features are non-specific and do not distinguish between different aetiologies. Similarly, the pattern of liver function test abnormality is non-specific.
- Timing and severity of graft dysfunction should guide further investigation (see Table 5.5).
- Severe graft dysfunction with prolonged INR and hyperlactataemia on the first postoperative day is highly suspicious for preservation injury or primary graft non-function.
- A marked transaminitis (AST >1000IU/L) in the first few days after transplant may be due to hepatic artery thrombosis and should be urgently investigated by duplex US and/or CT.
- Mild transaminitis in the early post-transplant period is often due to acute rejection, but may also be due to other causes (e.g. hepatitis C recurrence). Histological confirmation is essential before commencing anti-rejection therapy.
- Early graft recovery is indicated by AST <2000IU/L, INR <3, lactate <2mmol/L within 36h post-transplantation. In a patient with good

graft function, serum AST reduces by half each day until normal. A rise in AST may be due to:
- rejection;
- sepsis;
- vascular insult.

Table 5.5 Causes of graft dysfunction according to time after liver transplant

Early (up to 4 weeks)	Intermediate (up to 6 months)	Late (after 6 months)
Primary non-function	Acute rejection	Chronic rejection
Preservation injury	Technical complication	Disease recurrence
Technical complication	Disease recurrence (hepatitis B and C)	PTLD*
Acute rejection	CMV hepatitis	Drug-induced
Sepsis	EBV hepatitis	Biliary stricture
		Late HAT**

*Post-transplant lymphoproliferative disease.
**Hepatic artery thrombosis.

Investigation of graft dysfunction
- FBC, U&E, LFTs.
- INR.
- Arterial lactate.
- Duplex US +/– CT.
- MRCP +/– ERCP if suspected bile leak or stricture.
- Blood cultures if septic.
- CMV DNA titre.
- EBV serology.
- HBV serology.
- HCV RNA.
- Percutaneous liver biopsy.

Technical complications

Haemorrhage

- Exacerbated by coagulopathy/thrombocytopaenia and/or poor early graft function.
- **Potential sources:**
  - injury to donor liver during retrieval;
  - vascular anastomoses;
  - liver biopsy sites;
  - hepatic or splenic artery pseudoaneurysm (due to infection);
  - splenic rupture.
- Urgent reoperation if:
  - haemodynamic instability;
  - significant transfusion requirement;
  - abdominal compartment syndrome.
- If patient stable, arrange urgent CT angiography and correct coagulopathy/thrombocytopaenia.

Hepatic artery thrombosis

- Incidence 2–5% in adults, 4-8% in children (smaller vessels).
- Usually develop early (<10 days), but may occur late.
- **Risk factors:**
  - high resistance (small calibre vessels, multiple arteries, atheroma, intimal injury during handling);
  - poor inflow (high dose vasopressors, prolonged hypotension);
  - poor outflow (graft oedema due to dysfunction, IVC stenosis/obstruction);
  - prothrombotic states.
- **Clinical features:**
  - *Liver necrosis* – develops in early hepatic artery thrombosis (HAT). Quiescent in early phase, but patients may grow Gram –ive organisms on blood culture. Later features include significant transaminitis, coagulopathy, and/or shock.
  - *Liver abscesses* – presents 2–3 months post-transplant with fever/pain. Requires re-transplantation.
  - *Ischaemic cholangiopathy* – late HAT, presents with graft dysfunction and biliary strictures.
- **Diagnosis:** Duplex US and/or CT angiography.
- **Management:**
  - *Early HAT–*
    - thrombectomy +/– revision of arterial anastomosis if no evidence of necrosis on CT;
    - urgent re-transplantation.
  - *Late HAT –*
    - biliary reconstruction if biliary stricture confined to extrahepatic ducts;
    - re-transplantation.

Portal vein stenosis/thrombosis

- Incidence 2%.
- **Risk factors:**
  - previous portal vein thrombosis;
  - size mismatch;
  - large portosystemic collaterals (steal phenomenon);
  - kinking or torsion (due to excess length);
  - anastomostic stenosis.
- **Clinical features:**
  - early PV thrombosis → graft dysfunction, acute portal hypertension (ascites/variceal bleeding);
  - late PV thrombosis.
- **Diagnosis:** Duplex US +/− CT angiogram +/− portal pressure studies.
- **Management:**
  - *early PV thrombosis* – if diagnosed within 1–2 days, thrombectomy may be effective; if associated with graft failure, only option is re-transplantation;
  - *late PV stenosis* – angioplasty or surgical revision;
  - *late PV thrombosis* – treat complications of portal HT, consider TIPS if intrahepatic, consider shunt surgery. Re-transplantation if graft dysfunction.

Venous outflow obstruction

- Stenosis at the suprahepatic IVC anastomosis or hepatic veins if piggyback.
- Incidence 1–2%
- **Risk factors:**
  - anastomotic narrowing;
  - torsion of graft on venous pedicle;
  - mechanical obstruction by large graft;
  - recurrent Budd-Chiari syndrome.
- **Clinical features:** hepatomegaly, ascites, renal failure, graft dysfunction, bilateral leg swelling.
- **Diagnosis:** US/CT angiography or MRV.
- **Management:**
  - revisional surgery;
  - re-transplantation.

Bile leak

- Incidence 5–10%.
- Anastomotic:
  - technical;
  - ischaemia.
- Non-anastomotic:
  - aberrant ducts;
  - cut surface leaks (split or reduced grafts).
- **Management:** If persistent, ERCP +/− stent. If leak after bilio-enteric anastomosis, PTC +/− stent. Ensure adequate drainage of bilomas.

Biliary stricture

- Incidence 5–15%.
- **Anastomotic:**
  - Technical;
  - unrecognized bile leak;
  - covert ischaemia.
- **Non-anastomotic:**
  - primary sclerosing cholangitis;
  - hepatic artery thrombosis.
- Clinical features: graft dysfunction, jaundice, cholangitis, liver abscess (if associated with HAT).
- **Management:** drain biliary tree, treat sepsis, and obtain cholangiogram. Consider biliary reconstructive surgery (Roux-en-Y hepatico-jejunostomy). Retransplant if associated with HAT.

Infectious complications

Bacterial

- Early episodes (<1 week) often associated with line sepsis or graft dysfunction (*Staphylococcus aureus, Streptococcus* spp., *E. coli, Pseudomonas aeruginosa*).
- Less common organisms may cause late infections (e.g. *Legionella* spp., *Listeria monocytogenes, Mycobacterium* spp.).
- Alert organisms (MRSA, vancomycin-resistant enterococcus, *Streptococcus pyogenes, Clostridium difficile*).

Viral

- Tend to present >2 weeks.
- Cytomegalovirus infection (if donor CMV-positive and recipient CMV-negative) or reactivation (if recipient CMV-positive).
- Herpes simplex.
- Varicella zoster.
- Epstein-Barr virus.
- Hepatitis B re-infection.
- Hepatitis C re-infection.
- HIV.

Fungal

- Tend to present in second week post-transplant.
- Increased incidence in patients with acute liver failure, significant graft dysfunction, and after retransplant.
- *Candida* spp.
- *Aspergillus* spp.
- *Cryptococcus* spp.
- *Histoplasm* spp.
- *Pneumocystis carinii*.

Parasitic

Toxoplasma gondii.

Rejection

Hyperacute rejection
- Very rare after liver transplant.
- Preformed HLA antibodies cause complement-mediated damage to graft endothelium.
- Presents with rapid onset of liver failure.
- Treat by urgent re-transplantation.

Acute cellular rejection
- Common (30–50%).
- Presents with early graft dysfunction (rise in transaminases). Patient usually clinically well and asymptomatic. May be preceded by fever.
- Diagnosed by percutaneous liver biopsy.
- **Histological features** (2 of following):
  - portal tract inflammation (mixed infiltrate);
  - bile duct damage;
  - endothelitis.
- Banff grading system (mild, moderate or severe).
- Rejection activity index.
- **Management:**
  - pulsed steroids (1g methyprednisolone od. for 3 days);
  - monitor graft function – if persistent transaminitis, consider
    - optimizing immunosuppressant levels;
    - repeat pulsed steroids;
    - consider ATG or OKT3 if severe, steroid non-responsive rejection.

Chronic rejection
- Incidence <10%.
- **Risk factors:**
  - persistently low immunosuppressant levels;
  - acute rejection (multiple episodes, severe AR);
  - hepatitis C infection;
  - CMV mismatch.
- Presents with progressive cholestasis (predominant rise in GGT and ALP), followed by hyperbilirubinaemia.
- **Natural history:** early stages may be reversible with optimal immunosuppression, although re-transplantation may become necessary.
- Diagnosed by percutaneous liver biopsy.
- **Histological features:**
  - ductopenia (loss of interlobular bile ducts);
  - hepatocyte ballooning +/– necrosis in zone 3 of the hepatic lobule;
  - arteriopathy.
- **Management:** optimize immunosuppressant levels. Consider switching to Sirolimus. Re-transplant if progressive graft dysfunction.

Liver lesions

N. Battula, R. Sutcliffe, R. Deshpande, & O. Tucker

Cystic lesions

Non-neoplastic

Simple cyst

- Aberrant development of intrahepatic bile ducts. Do not usually communicate with the biliary ductal system (Fig. 6.1).
- Common (1–3% of routine liver scans).
- Sex preponderance: female > male.
- Can be solitary or multiple; variable size up to >20cm.
- Usually asymptomatic.
- Symptoms occur due to complications, e.g. bleeding, rupture, secondary infection, compression of adjacent structures (IVC, portal vein, bile ducts).
- Treat if symptomatic or if malignancy suspected.

Adult polycystic liver disease

- Autosomal dominant inheritance.
- Usually associated with polycystic kidney disease.
- Characterized by multiple, variable sized cysts ranging in size from several mm to ≥12cm (Fig. 6.2).
- Usually asymptomatic.
- Symptoms arise due to massive hepatomegaly, spontaneous haemorrhage, infection, rupture, liver dysfunction with liver failure (rare), biliary obstruction.
- Treat if symptomatic. Options include open/laparoscopic fenestration or resection. Combined liver and renal transplantation if associated with polycystc kidneys and end-stage renal failure.

Caroli's disease

- Congenital communicating ectasia of the biliary tree.
- Rare.
- Autosomal recessive inheritance.
- Affects large intrahepatic bile ducts.
- Segmental or diffuse distribution.
- Saccular or fusiform dilation of bile ducts occurs with stricture formation, multiple intrahepatic calculi, and recurrent attacks of cholangitis.
- Complications include recurrent ascending cholangitis and cholangiocarcinoma.
- **Caroli's syndrome** = Caroli's disease *plus* congenital hepatic fibrosis.

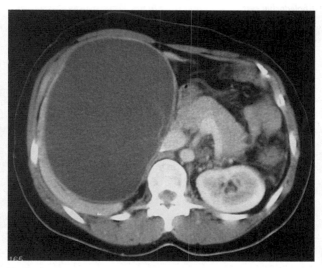

Fig. 6.1 Liver cyst.

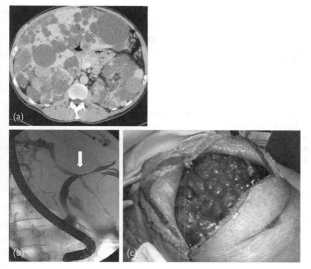

Fig. 6.2 (a–c) Polycystic liver disease. Image 2 is an ERCP of a patient with polycystic liver disease in whom a dominant cyst had caused obstructive jaundice due to compression of the hilar confluence (arrowed).

Choledochal cyst
- Rare congenital dilation of the hepatic duct (Fig. 6.3).
- Communicates with biliary tree.
- **Modani classification** (types 1 to 5): type 5 is also known as Caroli's disease.
- Symptoms due to complications, e.g. ascending cholangitis, CBD stones, abdominal mass, pancreatitis, cholangiocarcinoma.

Biliary hamartoma (Von Meyenburg complex)
- Failure of involution of embryonic bile ducts.
- Associated with congenital hepatic fibrosis and polycystic liver disease.
- Usually incidental finding at operation.
- Usually asymptomatic.
- No communication with biliary tree.

Infection
- Pyogenic abscess.
- Amoebic abscess.
- Fungal abscess.
- Hydatid cyst.

Trauma
- Intrahepatic haematoma.
- Subcapsular haematoma.
- Intrahepatic biloma.

Neoplastic

Biliary cystadenoma
- Rare, middle-aged women.
- Non-specific symptoms.
- **US/CT:** thick-walled or multiloculated cyst with solid components.
- **Differential diagnosis:** cystadenocarcinoma.
- Treatment is surgical resection.

Other cystic neoplasms
- Biliary cystadenocarcinoma.
- Cystic hepatocellular carcinoma.
- Central cystic degeneration in giant cavernous haemangioma (Fig. 6.4).
- Cystic metastases.
- Cystic malignant melanoma.
- Cystic neuroendocrine tumour.
- Cystic sarcoma.

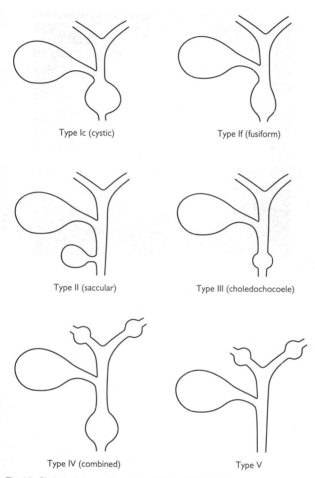

Fig. 6.3 Choledochal cysts. Type Ic (cystic). Type If (fusiform). Type II (saccular). Type III (choledochocoele). Type IV (combined). Type V.

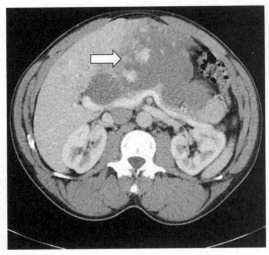

Fig. 6.4 Cavernous haemangioma (arrowed).

Liver abscesses

Causes

Local sepsis
- Cholangitis.
- Gangrenous cholecystitis.
- Ischaemic cholangiopathy (e.g. hepatic artery thrombosis post-liver transplant).
- Localized bile leak (post-liver resection or instrumentation, e.g. radio-frequency ablation).

Portal pyaemia
- Acute diverticulitis.
- Acute appendicitis.
- Acute pancreatitis.
- Amoebiasis.
- Hydatid disease.

Systemic sepsis
- Bacteraemia.
- Subacute bacterial endocarditis.

Differential diagnosis
Cystic tumour (e.g. cystic metastasis).

Clinical features
- Fevers, rigors, malaise, right upper quadrant pain, and tenderness.
- Jaundice if biliary obstruction.
- Abnormal LFTs, raised inflammatory markers.
- 25–30% of liver abscesses occur in diabetics and they may be the first presentation of the condition.

Investigations
- FBC, U&E, LFTs, INR.
- Fasting blood glucose and HbA1C.
- Blood cultures.
- US/CT to further characterize lesion(s) and evaluate for primary gastrointestinal sources of sepsis.
- MRCP/ERCP if suspected biliary obstruction, cholangiopathy, or bile leak.
- Consider gastroscopy or colonoscopy to exclude gastrointestinal pathology.
- Hydatid serology.
- Amoebic serology.
- Aspirate pus from abscess, *except* in patients with hydatid disease (❶ **risk of anaphylaxis**).

Pyogenic abscess
- Aspirate pus under US or CT guidance. If residual pus or evidence of bile leak, leave pigtail catheter *in situ* until dry.
- Broad-spectrum antibiotics, amended according to microbiology and sensitivities. Initially give IV, then convert to oral when patient systemically well. Continue for 6 weeks.
- Treat underlying cause.

Amoebic abscess

- *Entamoeba histolytica* is transmitted within cysts via the faeco-oral route and may lay dormant in the gastrointestinal tract for many years, before manifesting as amoebic dysentery and/or amoebic liver abscesses.
- Liver abscess presents with non-specific symptoms, malaise, fever, and pain. May also rupture and present with acute abdomen.
- Diagnosis should be confirmed by amoebic serology or, if negative, microbiological analysis of abscess fluid.
- First-line treatment is oral metronidazole.
- If no response after 72h, aspirate abscess to dryness.

Hydatid liver disease

Hydatid disease, hydatidosis, echinococcosis (Fig. 6.5).

Aetiology

Zoonosis caused by the larval stage of *Taenia echinococcus*.

Epidemiology

- Worldwide distribution.
- Endemic in Middle and Far East, East Africa, Australia, New Zealand, South America, and many Mediterranean countries.

Biology

Three species of *Taenia echinococcus* can cause disease:

Echinococcus granulosus

- Most common species causing disease in humans.
- **Definitive host:** domestic and wild dogs, foxes, and wolves.
- **Intermediate host:** sheep, swine, cow, camel, goat, buffalo, human.
- **Life cycle:** in the definitive host, the adult tapeworm, consisting of a head (scolex), neck and 3–5 segments, measuring 3–6mm in length, attaches to the ileal mucosal villi. The terminal segment (proglottis) contains male and female gonads with approximately 5000 eggs. Segmentation occurs with development of 6 hooked embryos (oncospheres or hexacanth embryos). The terminal proglottis detaches, disintegrates, and ova are passed in the faeces.
- Humans are an accidental intermediate host infected by direct contact with dogs, or indirectly via contaminated water, food, or objects.
- In the intermediate host, the embryophore is digested in the duodenum, and the released onchosphere penetrates the mucosa to enter the portal circulation.
- The larval stage with hydatid cyst formation proceeds within the liver in 80%, with involvement of any organ after hepatic venous invasion.
- **Primary echinococcosis:** complete sexual cycle involving both the definitive and intermediate host with development of the larval stage.
- **Secondary echinococcosis:** asexual cycle in the intermediate host where new hydatid cyst(s) arise from the larval stage.

Echinococcus multilocularis

- **Definitive host:** dog, cat, red and artic fox.
- **Intermediate host:** field mouse, lemming, field/red backed vole, human.
- Similar life cycle to *Echinococcus granulosus*.
- Rarely causes disease in humans.
- May result in alveolar echinococcosis, a potentially fatal disease, in the liver.

Echinococcus oligartus

- **Definitive host:** wild felines.
- **Intermediate host:** agoutis, human.
- Larval stage results in multilocular liver involvement.

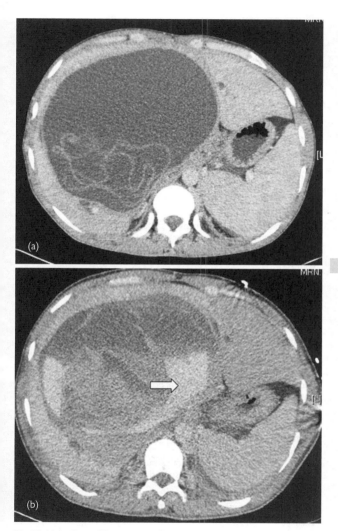

Fig. 6.5 Hydatid cyst. CT appearance of hydatid liver disease. (a) Ectocyst and endocyst clearly defined as two layers. (b) The presence of haemoperitoneum with active bleeding from the right portal vein (arrowed) due to rupture of a hydatid cyst into it.

Development of the hydatid cyst

If phagocytosis of the parasite fails to occur, a hydatid follicle is formed progressing to a hydatid cyst with the following elements:
- **Pericyst:** mainly avascular adventitial capsule of compressed and atrophic liver tissue.
- **Ectocyst or laminated membrane:** outer layer of cyst wall. Separated from the pericyst by narrow capillary space.
- **Endocyst or germinative membrane:** inner layer of cyst wall. Responsible for the production of hydatid fluid, brood capsules, protoscoleces and daughter cysts. Divided into 3 layers – tegument responsible for synthesis of the laminated membrane, tegumental cell region responsible for transport mechanism control, and an inner layer with absorptive and proliferative functions.
- **Hydatid sand:** brood capsules, protoscoleces (approximately 400,000/mL), and calcareous bodies within the hydatid cyst fluid.

Clinical features
- Asymptomatic.
- Symptomatic with development of complications:
  - right upper quadrant or lower chest pain;
  - abdominal fullness with hepatomegaly;
  - dyspepsia;
  - vomiting;
  - *weight loss* – 'Hydatid cachexia';
  - jaundice, pruritus;
  - urticarial rash, anaphyalaxis;
  - sympathetic pleural effusion for cysts located in the dome;
- **Rupture into the biliary tree:**
  - cystobiliary fistula;
  - *presentation* – biliary colic, cholestatic jaundice with recurrent ascending cholangitis, pyogenic abscess formation;
  - *diagnosis* – faecal passage of germinative membranes.
- **Rupture into the bronchial tree:** bronchobiliary fistula.
- Free rupture into the peritoneal, pleural or pericardial cavity.
- Rupture into adjacent organs, e.g. gallbladder, stomach, duodenum, aorta, IVC.

Indications for intervention
- Complicated cysts.
- Large, peripherally located, uncomplicated, viable cysts.
- Asymptomatic trauma-prone cysts in fit patients.

Contraindications to intervention
- Elderly unfit patients with small, asymptomatic, calcified cyst.
- Small deep cyst ≤4cm.

Intervention

Surgical

- Cyst decompression to ↓ intracystic pressure, drainage, daughter cyst evacuation, evaluation and management of cystobiliary fistula, ectocyst excision, scolecidal instillation using hypertonic saline (only if no biliary fistula present), residual cyst cavity obliteration by:
  - external drainage;
  - leaving cyst open to drain;
  - omentoplasty;
  - hepatic resection.
- Closed total cystopericystectomy.
- Open total cystopericystectomy.
- Non-anatomical liver resection.
- Anatomical liver resection.
- **Liver transplantation:** usually indicated for long-term complications (e.g. cholangiopathy secondary to scolecidal instillation).

Radiological drainage

- Percutaneous aspiration, injection (of scolecidal agent) and re-aspiration (PAIR) technique.

Medical management

Most effective for pulmonary hydatid disease.

Indications

- Perioperative treatment (2 weeks before surgery and 4 weeks postoperatively).
- Patients unfit for surgical intervention.
- Adjuvant therapy in those with intraoperative spillage.
- Following cyst rupture.
- Patients with widely disseminated hydatid disease.

Agents

- **Benzimidazole carbamates: mebendazole, albendazole:** mixed effectiveness against the larval stage of *Echinococcus granulosus* and *E. multilocularis*.
- **Praziquantel:** most effective agent for alveolar hydatidosis.

Problems

- Determining correct dose and duration of treatment.
- Identifying those patients with viable cysts only.
- Occurrence of spontaneous cyst resolution.

Benign tumours

Liver haemangioma
- Most common benign liver tumour.
- Prevalence in the general population 1–20%.
- F > M.
- Usually asymptomatic.
- Usually solitary, diameter ≤5cm.
- Diameter ≥10cm classified as giant haemangiomas.
- Natural history is variable – stable, involution or expansion.
- Malignant transformation to *angiosarcoma* extremely rare.
- **Symptoms:** pain, compression of adjacent structures, haemorrhage, rupture (+/– haemoperitoneum).
- Exclude haemangio-endothelioma (children) and haemangiopericytoma by MRI.
- Resect if symptomatic.

Focal nodular hyperplasia
- Prevalence in the general population 1–3% (Fig 10.3)
- Aetiology unknown. Possible hyperplastic response to pre-existing arteriovenous malformation. Possible role for OCP in aetiology.
- M = F.
- More frequent in women aged 30–50 years.
- Usually asymptomatic. Symptoms due to pain or compression of adjacent structures.
- Usually an incidental finding.
- **Type I (80%) 'typical':** lobulated, well circumscribed, solid, hypervascular lesion with a central scar containing large artery + multiple radiating fibrous septa.
- **Type II (20%) 'atypical':** heterogenous appearance with no central scar.
- No malignant potential.
- Withdraw OCP (if relevant) and review.
- Resect if symptomatic.

Hepatocellular adenoma
- Rare benign neoplasm of hepatocellular origin.
- More frequent in women aged 30–50 years.
- Solitary in 70–80%.
- Well circumscribed lesions ranging in size from 1 to >15cm diameter.
- **Risk factors:** long-term OCP or anabolic steroid use, type I glycogen storage disease, diabetes mellitus.
- Often regress with steroid withdrawal or blockade. Steroids may precipitate enlargement of a pre-existing adenoma and lead to complications.
- Usually asymptomatic. Symptoms include pain, haemorrhage, rupture.
- **Liver adenomatosis**: multiple hepatic adenomas, liver dysfunction, no association with anabolic steroid use, M = F, risk of HCC.
- Resect if symptomatic or >4cm.

Pseudo-lesions of the liver
- Focal fatty infiltration.
- Focal fatty sparing.
- Intrahepatic arterioportal shunts.
- Diaphragmatic parenchymal compression.
- Unenhanced vessels on dynamic imaging.
- Vascular abnormalities.
- Steal phenomenon around highly vascular lesions.

Malignant tumours

Primary malignancy in a cirrhotic liver
Hepatocellular carcinoma.

Primary malignancy in a non-cirrhotic liver
- **Hepatocyte origin:** hepatocellular carcinoma, fibrolamellar carcinoma, hepatoblastoma.
- **Bile duct origin:** cholangiocarcinoma, biliary cystadenocarcinoma.
- **Mesenchymal origin:** angiosarcoma, epithelioid haemangioendothelioma, lymphoma.

Investigation of liver lesions

Imaging techniques for segmental lesion localization
- **US:** transabdominal, contrast, intraoperative (open or laparoscopic).
- **CT:** dynamic spiral and multi-detector.
- **MRI**.

Diagnostic image-guided techniques
- Biopsy.
- Fine needle aspiration cytology.

Therapeutic image-guided techniques
- Radiofrequency ablation (RFA).
- Microwave ablation.
- Laser ablation.
- Cryotherapy.
- Transarterial chemoembolization (TACE).

Hepatocellular carcinoma

Epidemiology
- Fifth most common cancer worldwide.
- >80% of cases found in Africa or East Asia.
- Rising incidence in the West due to increasing incidence of viral hepatitis.
- Usually affects patients aged 50–70 years. Earlier onset (25–40 years) in Africa.
- M > F 2–4×.

Pathogenesis
- 70–90% of HCC develop on background of cirrhosis, particularly in relation to hepatitis B and C infection, alcohol, and haemochromatosis. In cirrhosis, HCC occurs due to chronic injury, regeneration, and dysplasia (Fig. 6.6).
- Hepatitis B virus is directly oncogenic and can cause HCC in the absence of cirrhosis.

Pathology
- Nodular or diffuse.
- Solitary or multifocal.
- **Fibrolamellar HCC:** a rare variant in non-cirrhotic livers of young adults. Less aggressive, but presents later with large mass, lymph node metastases, and normal AFP.
- Tumour differentiation and vascular invasion are important predictors of survival after surgical resection or liver transplantation.
- May rupture and bleed into peritoneal cavity, or spread via blood-stream leading to distant metastases in bone, lung, brain, adrenal glands.

Clinical presentation
- Asymptomatic, detected by routine US (e.g. screening in patients with cirrhosis).
- HCC may cause decompensation of chronic liver disease (e.g. due to portal vein thrombosis).
- Locally advanced disease may present with weight loss, anorexia, abdominal pain, and hepatomegaly.
- Ruptured HCC usually presents with peritonitis and shock.

Investigations
- Depends on mode of presentation.
- Aims of investigations are to:
  - confirm diagnosis of HCC radiologically;
  - determine extent of liver involvement;
  - exclude extrahepatic disease;
  - determine presence/absence of underlying liver disease (including viral status);
  - determine severity of liver disease.
- Serum alpha-foetoprotein is elevated in only 50–60% of cases, but is useful as a baseline prior to treatment.

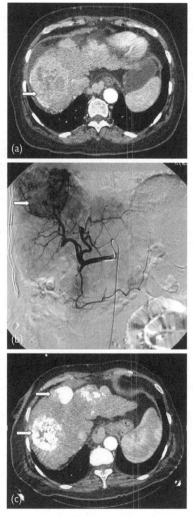

Fig. 6.6 Hepatocellular carcinoma. (a) Hepatocellular carcinoma in a patient with cirrhosis. (b) CT scans before and after transarterial chemoembolization. (c) Angiogram shows the vascular tumour prior to embolization.

- **Confirm diagnosis and determine extent of liver involvement.** US capable of detecting 2cm lesions, but further characterization by CT or MRI is necessary. HCC appears as hypervascular lesion with peripheral enhancement on triphasic CT or MRI with Tesla. Biopsy usually not indicated and is considered to carry a risk of tumour seeding along the needle track (1–2%).
- **Exclude extrahepatic disease.** CT chest +/– bone scan.
- **Underlying liver disease:** CT scan +/– biopsy of non-tumour liver if doubt.
- **Severity of liver disease:** Child-Pugh or MELD score.

Staging systems

- Several systems have been used, including TNM, Cancer of the Liver Italian Program (CLIP), Barcelona Clinic Liver Cancer (BCLC), Okuda and Japan Integrated Staging (JIS). Several factors have been incorporated into each system, and relate to tumour load and biology (size, number, presence of extrahepatic disease, and presence of vascular invasion), liver reserve (Child-Pugh score or its components), and performance status.
- Although these systems predict survival, they do not allow selection of patients for potentially curative treatment (resection or liver transplantation).
- In 1996, the *Milan criteria* were the first to be published that defined a subgroup of patients who were suitable for liver transplantation. Milan criteria are:
  - single HCC <5cm;
  - three tumours <3cm, in the absence of extrahepatic disease and vascular invasion.
- The expanded *UCSF criteria* were not associated with a reduced disease-free survival after liver transplantation. UCSF criteria are:
  - single HCC <6.5cm;
  - three tumours <4.5cm, in the absence of extrahepatic disease and vascular invasion.

Management

Localized disease

- **No cirrhosis or Child A cirrhosis:** resect if technically feasible. If unresectable, consider alternative local ablative therapies (TACE, RFA, PEI).
- **Child B/C cirrhosis:** liver transplantation if within Milan (or UCSF) criteria and no anaesthetic/surgical contraindications. Consider pre-transplant TACE or RFA in borderline cases *and* if predicted waiting time from listing to transplantation >7 months.

Unresectable or metastatic disease

- Palliative systemic chemotherapy (Doxorubicin).
- Sorafenib (tyrosine kinase inhibitor) significantly improves median survival in patients with advanced disease. Its role in an adjuvant setting is currently unknown.
- Palliative care.

Treatment modalities and outcomes

Liver resection

- **Indications:** absence of extrahepatic disease in a patient with no underlying liver disease or Child A cirrhosis.
- **Minor resections** may be considered in patients with early Child B without portal hypertension (hepatic vein pressure <10mmHg).
- **High risk of recurrence** in remnant liver (distant from resection margin).
- **5-year overall survival:** 25–60%.
- Disease-free survival is better after anatomical than non-anatomical resection (5-year 63% v. 35%).

Liver transplantation

- Allows radical resection of tumour and treatment of underlying liver disease.
- Excellent long-term disease-free post-transplant survival if restricting patients to Milan or UCSF criteria.
- 30% of patients will exceed Milan criteria on histological examination of the explanted liver, and adverse histological features (multifocal disease, vascular invasion, and poorly differentiated tumours) carry a poor prognosis.
- Pre-transplant tumour biopsy is recommended by a few centres in order to incorporate tumour histology into selection of patients for transplant in addition to size criteria. Anecdotal reports of tumour seeding along needle biopsy tracks have prevented this approach from becoming standard practice.
- Cadaveric organ shortage is a major factor that limits the role of liver transplantation for HCC. Live donor liver transplantation is an alternative, but this approach is hindered by the risks of donor morbidity and mortality.

Tumour ablation

- PEI and RFA suitable for tumours <4cm in patients unfit for surgery.
- Tumour ablation occurs in >90%.
- No RCTs comparing PEI or RFA with liver resection.

TACE

- Safe and effective measure to control tumour progression (40% response rate) prior to liver transplantation, for patients fulfilling Milan criteria.
- Response rate to TACE may predict disease-free survival after liver transplantation.

Cholangiocarcinoma

Epidemiology
- Uncommon; 2% of all malignancies.
- Increased incidence in Far East.
- Peak incidence in 70's.
- M > F.

Types
- **Extrahepatic** (90%): 2/3 arise at the hilar confluence ('Klatskin tumours' or *hilar cholangiocarcinoma*); 1/3 arise in distal bile duct (*distal cholangiocarcinoma*; Fig. 6.7).
- **Intrahepatic** (10%): also known as *peripheral cholangiocarcinoma*.

Aetiology
- Majority are sporadic.
- **Risk factors:** PSC, congenital biliary disease (choledochal anomaly, (10–30% risk), liver fluke (*Clonorchis sinensis*), oriental cholangiohepatitis, aflatoxins, vinyl chloride, thorotrast, nitrosamines, benign biliary tumours (papilloma and adenoma).
- *PSC and cholangiocarcinoma*: lifetime risk 5–15%. Incidence of CC is 1.5% per year (highest risk in first 2 years of diagnosis).

Pathology
- Majority are adenocarcinoma. Rarely, squamous cell carcinoma, small cell, and papillary.
- Usually associated with intense fibrotic reaction.
- Spreads longitudinally along biliary tree.
- Lymph node involvement at presentation is common and carries a poor prognosis. **NB.** Enlarged lymph nodes may be inflammatory and must be biopsied.
- Haematogenous spread is uncommon.

Classification
- **Bismuth classification:**
  - *Type I* – below the hilar confluence;
  - *Type II* – at the confluence;
  - *Type III* – extending into first order right (IIIa) or left (IIIb) ducts;
  - *Type IV* – bilateral second order duct involvement.
- **TNM staging:**
  - *T1* – confined to mucosa;
  - *T2* – invading muscle;
  - *T3* – invading adjacent organs (liver, gallbladder, stomach);
  - *N1* – hilar lymph nodes;
  - *N2* – regional lymph nodes;
  - *M1* – distant metastases.

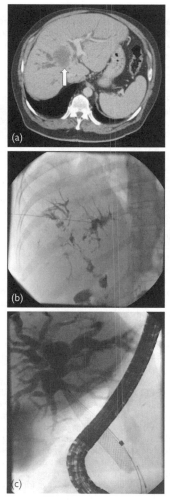

Fig. 6.7 Hilar cholangiocarcinoma. (a) Hilar cholangiocarcinoma arising from right hepatic duct, causing right-sided biliary dilatation. (b) Percutaneous cholangiogram of a locally advanced hilar cholangiocarcinoma with disconnection between left and right ducts. (c) Insertion of an expandable metallic stent into the common hepatic duct to palliate biliary obstruction in a patient with unresectable cholangiocarcinoma.

Clinical features
- **Obstructive jaundice:** hilar and distal cholangiocarcinoma.
- **Incidental finding on US/CT:** peripheral cholangiocarcinoma.
- **Non-specific symptoms:** weight loss, abdominal pain.
- Abnormal serum ALP and GGT.

Investigations
- LFTs.
- Raised CA-19.9 and CEA.
- **US:** dilated biliary tree to the level of tumour.
- **CT:** hilar mass, lymph node involvement, liver metastases, vascular involvement, portal vein occlusion, lobar atrophy (due to biliary obstruction).
- **MRI/MRCP:** defines the anatomical location of the tumour. Combine with MRA to assess contralateral vascular involvement.
- **ERCP:** useful for *distal cholangiocarcinoma* for assessing extent of tumour and obtaining biliary stenting.
- **PTC:** necessary for *hilar cholangiocarcinoma* to delineate anatomy and achieve external biliary drainage. Bilateral drains required if left and right ducts are disconnected.
- **Routine preoperative biliary drainage:** increased risk of postoperative infective complications, but should be performed prior to extended liver resection, or if cholangitis/renal failure.
- **Preoperative biopsy:** not routinely indicated, unless considering systemic chemotherapy.
- **Staging laparoscopy +/– laparoscopic US:** may improve the accuracy of pre-operative staging (diagnosis of peritoneal disease), thereby reducing rate of non-therapeutic laparotomy.

Management
Surgical resection
- Accurate preoperative staging.
- Treat sepsis/renal failure.
- Preoperative biliary drainage of the future liver remnant (FLR).
- **Assess volume of FLR:** consider preoperative contralateral portal vein embolization (PVE) to stimulate FLR hypertrophy (re-CT in 4–6 weeks to assess response prior to surgery). If planning PVE, need to perform bilobar biliary drainage first.
- Perform extended right or left hepatectomy (depending on preoperative imaging) with routine caudate resection and lymphadenectomy for *hilar cholangiocarcinoma*. Resect and reconstruct portal vein if indicated to achieve R0 resection. Send proximal and distal bile duct margins for frozen section analysis. If distal margin positive for tumour, perform simultaneous Whipple's pancreatico-duodenectomy. If negative, perform retrocolic Roux-en-Y hepatico-jejunostomy.
- Postoperative complications: liver failure (small-for-size syndrome), sepsis, bile leak. Operative mortality 5–10%.
- Predictors of survival are positive resection margins and lymph node involvement. 5-year overall survival 35–40% if R0 resection and node-negative disease.

- *Distal cholangiocarcinoma* should be treated by pancreatico-duodenectomy. *Peripheral (intrahepatic)* cholangiocarcinoma should be treated by anatomical liver resection.

Liver transplantation

- Locally advanced disease with vascular involvement precludes R0 resection in many patients with *hilar cholangiocarcinoma*.
- Liver transplantation may be an option in these patients, but for it to be accepted, 5-year survival figures must be comparable with those for other indications for liver transplant, given the ongoing cadaveric organ shortage.
- Most series report poor long-term survival after liver transplantation for cholangiocarcinoma, presumably due to occult metastases at the time of the procedure.
- The Mayo Clinic have published a large series of patients transplanted for node-negative cholangiocarcinoma with an impressive 5-year survival of 82%. All patients received pre-transplant chemoradiotherapy. This data has not yet been reproduced and, at present, cholangiocarcinoma is not an indication for liver transplantation in UK or Europe.
  In addition, there are concerns that pre-transplant radiotherapy significantly increases post-transplant morbidity.

Palliative treatment

- Self-expanding metallic stents have superior results to plastic stents for relief of jaundice in unresectable cases.
- Stents may be inserted either endoscopically or percutaneously.
- **Stent-related complications** include cholangitis, tumour in-growth, bleeding.
- **Palliative segment III bypass** may be indicated if stenting fails or in patients with a longer life expectancy.
- **Photodynamic therapy:** IV injection of a photosensitizer (e.g. Photofrin) followed by laser application (via ERCP or PTC). Activation causes release of free radicals leading to tumour cell lysis. Should be undertaken after metallic stent insertion. RCTs have demonstrated prolongation of median survival.
- There is currently no established role for chemotherapy or radiotherapy.

Colorectal liver metastases

Background

- Up to 70% of patients with colorectal cancer develop liver metastases.
- Untreated, patients with colorectal liver metastases (CLM) have a poor prognosis. Resection of CLM is associated with a significantly improved 5-year survival (50%), although no RCTs have been performed (see Fig. 6.8).
- Metastatic tumour cells enter the portal circulation, embolize in the liver parenchyma and develop into metastatic deposits.
- CLM may be present at the time of diagnosis of the colorectal primary tumour (*synchronous* metastasis) or may develop later (*metachronous* metastasis).
- In selected cases, 5-year survival after resection of colorectal liver metastases is 40%.

Diagnosis

- Usually asymptomatic, and found during staging of primary or on follow-up imaging. Rarely, advanced CLM may present with malaise, weight loss, and jaundice.
- Routine vs. intensive follow-up after colorectal cancer surgery. Currently, the subject of a UK RCT. It is not clear whether intensive follow-up with frequent US/CT improves the long-term survival of patients who develop CLM. Any observed survival benefit may be due to lead-time bias.
- After initial diagnosis on US or CT, MRI may be useful to determine volume and distribution of liver involvement, prior to deciding treatment. PET scan should be considered in patients being evaluated for potentially curative liver resection in order to exclude extrahepatic disease.

Principles of management

- The aim of any liver-directed treatment (e.g. surgical resection) should be to safely remove all viable tumour with a clear margin (>1cm). Intra-operative US should be used routinely to aid planning at the time of resection.
- Unresectable unilobar disease may be treated by neoadjuvant chemotherapy followed by extended liver resection (+/– portal vein embolization depending on the size of future liver remnant).
- In the presence of bilobar disease, clearance may be achieved by staged resections or a combination of resection and RFA.
- In the presence of synchronous, resectable lung metastases, clearance of the liver lesions should be undertaken first.
- Minor liver resections (two segments or less) may be safely performed at the same time as colorectal resection (open or laparoscopic). Major liver resections should be deferred until after the patient has recovered from colorectal surgery +/– adjuvant chemotherapy, particularly in the presence of comorbidity.

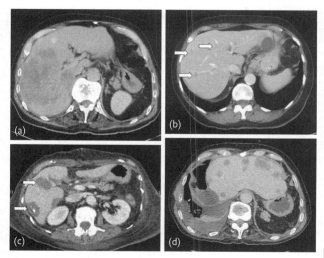

Fig. 6.8 Colorectal liver metastases. (a) Large solitary colorectal liver metastasis. (b, c) Multifocal liver metastases before and after radio-frequency ablation. (d) Recurrence of colorectal metastases in left lobe after previous right hepatectomy.

- Neoadjuvant or adjuvant oxaliplatin or irinotecan-based chemotherapy regimens should be considered in all patients undergoing treatment of colorectal liver metastases.
- The extent of liver resection should be determined by pre-chemotherapy imaging (CT or MRI) *not* post-chemotherapy imaging.
- Recurrent liver metastases after resection should be re-resected if technically feasible (similar long-term survival compared to first liver resection). Third time resections may also provide long-term benefit.

Liver resection vs. radiofrequency thermal ablation

- There have been no RCTs to date comparing liver resection with RFA for treatment of CLM.
- Based on the available evidence, liver resection is the preferred option for treating resectable CLM.
- RFA may be administered percutaneously or at operation (laparoscopic or open). The effect of RFA depends on tumour size, accessibility of the lesion, and proximity to major vessels or bile ducts.
- RFA may be employed in isolation in patients unfit for surgery, or as an adjunct to resection in patients with bilobar disease.

Neuroendocrine liver metastases

Background
- Heterogeneous group of rare tumours arising from neuroendocrine cells in the gastro-enteropancreatic system.
- Primary neuroendocrine tumours (NET) usually orginate in the gastrointestinal or respiratory tracts. Primary hepatic neuroendocrine tumours are extremely rare.
- Pancreatic NET may be part of multiple endocrine neoplasia syndrome type I or von Hippel Lindau syndrome.
- Peak incidence 30–60 years.
- M = F.

Pathology
- Slow growing.
- Functioning (hormone secretion) or non-functioning.
- Liver metastases common at time of diagnosis (75%).
- Most common histological types are *gastrinomas*, *carcinoid tumours* and *insulinomas*.
- Classified according to size, hormone production and histological appearance (see Table 6.1).

Table 6.1 Classification of neuroendocrine tumours

Grade I	Well-differentiated tumour confined to organ/mucosa (functioning or non-functioning)	Benign behaviour[1]
Grade II	Well-differentiated tumour confined to organ/mucosa (functioning or non-functioning)	Uncertain behaviour[2]
Grade III	Well-differentiated carcinoma (functioning or non-functioning)	Low-grade malignant with invasion +/– metastases
Grade IV	Poorly differentiated carcinoma (functioning or non-functioning)	High-grade malignant

[1]Benign behaviour is diameter <1cm (stomach or small intestine) or <2cm (pancreas, appendix, colon or rectum).

[2]Uncertain behaviour is diameter >1cm (stomach or small intestine) or >2cm (pancreas, appendix, colon or rectum).

Clinical features
- Usually asymptomatic until late. Symptoms due to:
  - compression of adjacent structures;
  - liver metastases;
  - hormone production (see Table 6.2).
- *Carcinoid syndrome* occurs due to secretion of 5-hydroxytryptamine (5-HT) by carcinoid liver metastases. Primary carcinoid tumours are clinically silent because 5-HT enters the portal circulation and is metabolized by the liver.

Table 6.2 Neuroendocrine clinical syndromes

Tumour	Hormone secreted	Syndrome
Insulinoma	Insulin	Hypoglycaemia, plasma glucose <3mM, symptoms relieved by glucose (Whipple's triad)
Gastrinoma	Gastrin	Zollinger-Ellison syndrome: recurrent peptic ulceration, diarrhoea, and malabsoprtion
VIPoma	Vasoactive polypeptide	Verner-Morrison syndrome: watery diarrhoea, hypokalaemia, achlorhydria
Glucagonoma	Glucagon	Necrolytic migratory erythema, glucose intolerance, weight loss, diarrhoea, DVT
Somatostatinoma	Somatostatin	Abdominal pain, diarrhoea, hyperglycaemia, gallstones
Carcinoid tumour	5-HT	Carcinoid syndrome: facial flushing, bronchospasm and profound hypotension

Diagnosis

- Non-functioning tumours usually diagnosed by histological analysis (e.g. after appendicectomy).
- Serum chromogranin A (secreted by majority of functioning and non-functioning tumours).
- Serum *gut hormone profile:* gastrin, VIP, somatostatin, glucagon.
- 24h urinary 5-hydroxy-indoleacetic acid (5-HIAA) to diagnose carcinoid syndrome.
- Fasting insulin and glucose levels to diagnose insulinoma.
- Localize primary tumour by somatostatin receptor scintigraphy (octreotide scan) or MIBG scan combined with cross-sectional imaging (CT, MRI, or EUS; Figs 6.9 and 6.10).
- Evaluate liver metastases using CT or MRI.
- Histological confirmation of diagnosis is only required if unresectable.

Management

Primary tumour
- Resect if possible.
- Acid suppression (proton pump inhibitors) for unresectable gastrinomas.

Resectable liver metastases
Liver resection.

Unresectable liver metastases
- Systemic therapy with somatostatin analogues (octreotide or lanreotide) for carcinoid syndrome.
- MIBG (metaiodobenzylguanidine) therapy (MIBG receptors over-expressed by 50% of NET).

- Debulking liver resection.
- Tumour ablation (chemoembolization or radiofrequency ablation).
- **Liver transplantation**: rarely performed now. Consider if no extrahepatic disease and biologically favourable histology (e.g. carcinoid).

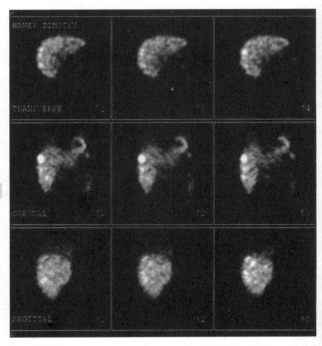

Fig. 6.9 MIBG scan showing uptake in a neuroendocrine liver metastasis.

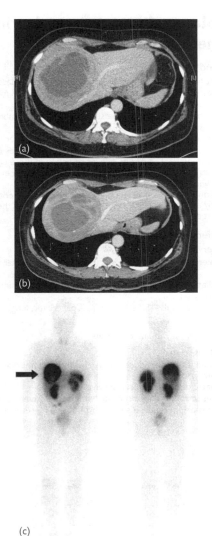

Fig. 6.10 Neuroendocrine liver metastases. (a,b) Large neuroendocrine liver metastasis in right lobe before and after right portal vein embolization to allow hypertrophy of left lobe prior to resection. (c) Appearances of tumour on octreotide scan.

Non-colorectal non-neuroendocrine liver metastases

Background

- In contrast to colorectal and neuroendocrine liver metastases, the value of resecting liver metastases from other solid organ malignancies is less well defined.
- Evidence is based on retrospective series, which have combined data from different primary tumours.
- Except for oesophageal, gastric, and pancreatic cancer, liver metastases from other primary sites occur due to systemic metastases (rather than portal venous). The results of liver resection in these cases is therefore influenced by the synchronous presence/absence of metastases elsewhere (i.e. extrahepatic disease).
- The decision to offer liver resection for this group of patients should be made by a multidisciplinary team, and take into account the following factors that affect survival after resection.

Factors affecting survival after liver resection

Site of primary tumour
- **Favourable:** 5-year survival 30–50% (ovarian, uterine, renal, testicular, breast).
- **Intermediate:** 5-year survival 15–30% (stomach, duodenum, melanoma).
- **Poor:** 5-year survival <15% (oesophageal, pancreatic, lung).

Patient-related
Age: reduced survival with increasing age.

Liver metastasis-related
- **Disease-free interval:** reduced survival with short interval (<12 months).
- **Extrahepatic disease:** reduced survival.
- **Type of resection:** reduced survival with major vs. limited resection.
- **Resection margin:** reduced survival with R1 vs. R0 resection.

Liver resection techniques

O. Tucker & R. Deshpande

Principles

Indications
- Symptomatic benign tumours or cysts.
- Suspected/known primary liver malignancy.
- Liver metastases (selected cases).

Incisions
- Bilateral subcostal incison. From tip of the right 10th rib 2cm below the costal margin to the lateral border of the left rectus abdominis.
- Bilateral subcostal with Mercedes incision. Upper midline extension is added to a bilateral subcostal incision to improve access to the suprahepatic IVC and hepatic veins. Risk of postoperative incisional hernia at the junction of the midline and subcostal wounds.
- J shaped. Midline laparotomy to approximately 2–3cm above the umbilicus curving slightly to extend horizontally to the level of the 10th rib (less postoperative pain with improved mobility).
- Laparoscopic. Port-site placement determined by site of pathology and type of resection. Additional use of hand-port to facilitate retraction.

Minimize blood loss
- Maintain low CVP (0–5cm H_2O).
- Restrict fluid replacement.
- Epidural anaesthetic.
- Vascular isolation techniques.

Avoid air emboli
- 15° Trendelenberg position.
- Careful surgical technique.

Resection margin
- Resection of normal liver should be minimized if resecting for benign disease.
- Aim for 1cm tumour-free margin for malignant tumours.
- Accept closer margin (2–3mm), if tumour close to vital structures (e.g. inferior vena cava).
- Resect adjacent organ (e.g. diaphragm) if possible and necessary to achieve R0 resection.

See Fig. 7.1.

Intraoperative ultrasound
- Confirm site of pathology.
- Detect additional lesions not present on preoperative imaging in 10–50%.
- Delineate vascular anatomy in relation to tumour.
- Identify adequacy of resection margins.
- Facilitate parenchymal-sparing resection.

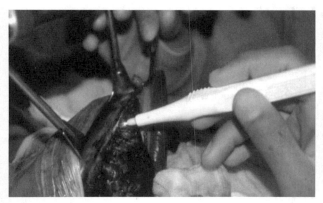

Fig. 7.1 Argon beam coagulation.

Parenchymal transection
- **Crush technique (or finger fracture):** crush liver parenchyma by repeated application of small straight haemostat. Fibrovascular stroma is left behind and cauterized using diathermy or argon beam coagulation, or divided between 4/0 vicryl ligatures or ligaclips.
- **Ultrasonic dissection with Cavitron Ultrasonic Surgical Aspirator (CUSA):** metal tip vibrates ultrasonically and shatters liver parenchyma. Liver tissue is then irrigated and aspirated with continuous high pressure suction. Blood vessels and biliary radicles are cauterized or ligated as above.
- **Water-jet dissection:** high pressure water jet shatters the liver parenchyma.
- **Harmonic scalpel:** ultrasonic energy is applied between tips of the forceps to seal blood vessels and transect parenchyma.
- **'Ligasure' device:** insulated metal-tip jaw crushes the parenchyma, revealing skeletonized vessels that can be coagulated and divided in a single application.
- **Vascular stapler.**

Haemostatic techniques
- Diathermy for vessels <3mm diameter.
- Suture ligation (3/0 or 4/0 prolene).
- Argon beam coagulation.
- Tissue glue (Tisseel, Bioglue).
- Haemostatic agents (Surgicel, Nu-knit).

Avoid torsion of liver remnant
- Essential to adequately fix liver remnant after right/extended right hepatectomy to prevent torsion and venous outflow obstruction.
- Re-suture falciform ligament to diaphragm/anterior abdominal wall.

Indications

Benign disease
- Adenoma.
- Cystadenoma.
- Haemangioma.
- Focal nodular hyperplasia (FNH).
- Liver cysts/polycystic liver disease.
- Caroli's disease.
- Intrahepatic gallstones.
- Intrahepatic strictures.
- Recurrent pyogenic cholangitis.
- Liver trauma.

Malignancy

Primary
- Hepatocellular carcinoma.
- Cholangiocarcinoma.
- Gallbladder carcinoma.

Metastatic
- Colorectal.
- Neuroendocrine.
- Non-colorectal non-neuroendocrine (malignant melanoma, breast, renal, endocrine, anal, genitourinary, sarcoma). Direct invasion of tumours in adjacent organs (adrenal, renal, gastric, colon, retroperitoneal sarcoma).

Preoperative assessment

Resectability
- Depends on the extent of liver pathology, number/distribution of lesions, proximity to major vascular structures, absence of extrahepatic disease.
- Criteria for resectability include:
  - clear radiological margin;
  - no residual lesion after surgery;
  - preservation of at least one hepatic vein and ipsilateral portal vein;
  - *adequate future liver remnant* – normal liver 20%, fatty liver 30–40%, Child's A cirrhosis 70%, Child's B cirrhosis 90%.

Types of resections
- Major anatomical vs. limited resection: reduced recurrence rate and improved survival.
- Segmental.
- Non-segmental:
  - wedge resection;
  - non-anatomical resection.
- Combination.

See Table 7.1.

Table 7.1 Types of hepatic resections

Segments resected	Couinaud (1957)	Goldsmith & Woodburne (1957)	Starzl (1982)
II, III, IV	L hepatectomy	L hepatic lobectomy	
II, III	L lobectomy	L lateral segmentectomy	
V, VI, VII, VIII	R hepatectomy	R hepatic lobectomy	
IV, V, VI, VII, VIII ± I	R lobectomy	Extended R hepatic lobectomy	R trisegmentectomy
II, III, IV, V, VIII ± I	Extended L hepatectomy	Extended L lobectomy	L trisegmentectomy

Vascular isolation

General approach

For segmental resections, the in-flow vessels (portal vein and hepatic artery) to the ipsilateral lobe may be isolated by extrahepatic or intrahepatic techniques:

- *Extrahepatic* – isolate ipsilateral portal pedicle and individually suture ligate portal vein and hepatic artery prior to parenchymal transection.
- *Intrahepatic* – perform hepatotomy, isolate and divide portal pedicle *en masse* prior to parenchymal transection (anterior or posterior Glissonian technique).
- *Combined approach* – extrahepatic dissection and temporary pedicle clamp occlusion, followed by isolation of major structures within liver during parenchymal transection.

Aims

- To ↓ intraoperative blood loss.
- To optimize patient haemodynamics.
- To avoid air embolism.
- To allow optimal surgical precision in a bloodless operative field.

Background

- Excessive blood loss is associated with ↑ perioperative morbidity and mortality.
- Perioperative blood transfusion may be associated with ↑ risk of recurrence and ↓ survival after resection for hepatobiliary malignancy by impairment of the immune system.
- The volume of perioperative blood transfused is an independent prognostic factor adversely effecting disease-free and overall survival after resection for colorectal liver metastases.
- Advances in liver resection techniques, with improved methods of vascular control and segmental-based surgical resections over the last 2 decades have reduced operative mortality to 2–4% in most large series.

Anatomical considerations

- The liver receives a dual blood supply from the portal vein (PV) (75%) and the hepatic artery (HA) (25%).
- Hepatic blood flow is 1500mL/min (25% of cardiac output).
- The HA provides 50% of the oxygen to the liver.
- The PV is formed behind the neck of the pancreas at the confluence of the superior mesenteric and splenic veins, travels posterior to the HA and bile duct (BD) in the free edge of the lesser omentum to the hilum where it divides into the right (RPV) and left PV (LPV).
- The LPV has a longer and more horizontal path compared to the right. Access to the RPV is therefore more difficult.
- The common HA arises from the coeliac axis, giving rise to the gastroduodenal and right gastric arteries to become the proper hepatic artery, passing superiorly on the medial aspect of the bile duct anterior to the PV, dividing at the hilum posterior to the bile ducts to form the RHA and LHA.

- The classical anatomical arrangements exist in only 50% of patients.
- An accessory or replaced LHA can arise from the left gastric artery to supply the left lobe, traversing the gastrohepatic omentum.
- An accessory or replaced RHA can arise from the superior mesenteric artery, passing to the hilum posterior to the PV.
- The liver is drained by the right, middle, left, and right inferior hepatic veins. A number of additional veins drain directly into the IVC from the caudate and posterior right lobe.
- Patients who have undergone prior abdominal operations may have extensive vascular adhesions in the right upper quadrant providing additional sources for blood loss if not adequately divided.

Techniques for vascular isolation

Selection of technique
Depends on:
- Indication for surgery, e.g. trauma vs. elective resection.
- Site of pathology.
- Extent of resection.
- **Patient factors:** haemodynamic status, cardiorespiratory comorbidity, diabetes.
- **Condition of the liver:** normal vs. fatty vs. fibrosis vs. cirrhosis.
- Experience of the surgeon.

Techniques
- **Inflow vascular control:** Pringle manoeuvre, hemihepatic vascular occlusion, segmental vascular occlusion.
- **Inflow and outflow vascular control:** total vascular isolation (TVI), inflow and extraparenchymal major hepatic vein occlusion.

Pringle manoeuvre

- First described in 1908 by J. Hogarth Pringle (Glasgow Royal Infirmary).
- Interruption of arterial and venous inflow to the liver by HA and PV occlusion.
- **Haemodynamic effects:** 10% increase in mean arterial pressure, 40% increase in systemic vascular resistance, 5% reduction in pulmonary artery pressure, 10% reduction in cardiac index.
- Initial inflow occlusion protects liver from subsequent periods of ischaemia (see Box 7.1).
- Divide adhesions to gain access to gastrohepatic ligament and hepatic hilum.
- Divide gastrohepatic ligament (avoiding injury to an accessory left HA).
- Pass an index finger behind the hilum through the foramen of Winslow and occlude the hilum using nylon tape or non-crushing clamp.
- Avoid excess occlusion to prevent arterial and biliary tree injury.
- Simultaneously occlude an accessory LHA if present.
- Pringle manoeuvre can be tolerated for 60min in a normal liver and 30min in a cirrhotic liver.
- Intermittent Pringle manoeuvre (repeated cycles of 10–20min clamping followed by 5min unclamping) increases the maximal period of clamping to 120min (or 45min in cirrhotic livers), improves

intraoperative haemodynamics, reduces vasopressor requirements post-reperfusion, and improves postoperative liver function.

Box 7.1 Ischaemic preconditioning

Technique
- Occlude liver inflow (portal vein and hepatic artery) for 5min.
- Restore inflow for 10min.
- Repeat 1 and 2.

Benefits
Protects liver from subsequent periods of ischaemia during parenchymal transection.

Side effects
May cause sudden release of anaerobic metabolites, lactic acid, and free radicals, leading to catastrophic haemodynamic collapse ('post-reperfusion injury'), particularly in patients with hepatic steatosis or chemotherapy-associated steatohepatitis (CASH).

Hemihepatic vascular isolation
- First described by Bismuth (1989).
- Selective vascular control to a single lobe allows demarcation of the line of parenchymal transection, and minimizes warm ischaemia of the future liver remnant.
- Perform cholecystectomy and ligate the cystic duct and cystic artery.
- Isolate the hepatoduodenal ligament and sling with nylon tape.
- Dissect the PV from right posterolateral aspect to hilar bifurcation, retracting the CHD medially. Encircle the PV retract laterally.
- Isolate RHA, encircle and retract medially.
- Isolate ipsilateral PV and occlude/divide.
- Isolate ipsilateral HA and occlude/divide.

Longmire clamping
- Allows vascular occlusion of a lobe without the Pringle manoeuvre.
- After lobe mobilization, a Longmire parenchymal compression clamp is placed across the lobe.
- Selective ligation of the lobar PV and HA can be performed for lobar resections.
- Segmental or wedge resections are possible by placing a smaller volume of parenchyma within the clamp.

Segmental vascular occlusion
- Interrupts the arterial and portal venous inflow to a liver segment.
- Dissect the segmental branch of the HA, encircle and clamp it.
- Identify the segmental branch of PV with a needle and syringe. Pass a flexible guide wire into the vessel and occlude it using a balloon catheter.
- Inject methylene blue into the segmental PV branch to confirm that supplies the appropriate segment.

Inflow and outflow occlusion

Total vascular isolation

- Described with (Heaney 1966) or without (Bismuth 1989) occlusion of the supracoeliac aorta.
- Complete isolation of the liver from the circulation.
- Allows safe resection of large tumours located close to hilar structures, hepatic veins, or IVC.
- TVI reduces blood loss, allows maximal parenchymal sparing.
- Can be tolerated for 60min in a normal liver under normothermic conditions. Hypothermic perfusion extends it to 90min.
- **Haemodynamic effects:** 50% rise in HR, 10% fall in systolic BP, 80% rise in SVR, 25% fall in pulmonary artery pressure, 40% fall in cardiac index.
- Poorly tolerated in 10–15% of patients. May cause major haemodynamic disturbance, requiring aggressive circulation support.
- **Technique:**
  - fully mobilize the liver, dividing all peritoneal attachments;
  - mobilize and encircle the IVC above and below the liver;
  - divide the right adrenal vein;
  - perform a Pringle manoeuvre;
  - trial clamp ×5min. Remove if >50% fall in CO or 30% fall in MAP;
  - *order of clamping* – (1) Pringle, (2) infrahepatic IVC, (3) suprahepatic IVC.
  - *order of unclamping* – (1) suprahepatic IVC, (2) infrahepatic IVC, (3) Pringle.

Inflow and extrahepatic hepatic vein occlusion

- Also called *hepatic vascular exclusion with preservation of caval flow* (HVEPC).
- Avoids IVC occlusion
- Described in 1995 by Elias.
- Risk of major haemorrhage with HV injury and air embolism.
- **Total vs. partial:** occlusion of all 3 HVs or single HV draining the lobe to be resected.
- **Control of RHV:**
  - divide falciform ligament to expose suprahepatic IVC and confluence of major HVs;
  - mobilize right lobe off IVC (including division of hepatocaval ligament);
  - expose and encircle RHV.

- **Control of LHV and MHV:**
  - mobilize left lobe;
  - divide peritoneal attachments above the caudate lobe to expose the LHV/IVC junction.

Further information

Bismuth, H., Castaing, D., & Garden, O.J. (1989) Major hepatic resection under total vascular exclusion. *Ann Surg* **210**, 13–19.

Heaney, J.P., Stanton, W.K., Halbert. D.S., Seidel, J., & Vice, T. (1966) An improved technique for vascular isolation of the liver: experimental study and case reports. *Ann Surg* **163**, 237–41.

Left hepatectomy

Mobilize left lobe

- Bilateral subcostal or J shaped incision.
- Adequate costal retraction.
- Perform IOUS to confirm the anatomical location of the tumour, identify additional tumours, and define the anatomical configuration of the major hepatic veins and portal pedicles.
- **Inflow occlusion:** intermittent Pringle manoeuvre.
- Divide and ligate the ligamentum teres (round ligament). Leave a long ligature on the divided ligamentum for later retraction.
- Divide the falciform ligament and separate from the upper anterior abdominal wall.
- Perform *en bloc* resection of the diaphragm if involved by tumour. Repair the defect with continuous non-absorbable suture.
- Place a swab behind the left lobe in front of the stomach. Using diathermy, divide the left triangular ligament from its tip to the medial margin of the suprahepatic IVC, mobilizing the left lobe from the diaphragm.
- Expose the anterior surface of the suprahepatic IVC at the level of the major hepatic vein confluence, staying close to the liver capsule.
- Divide the peritoneum over the left surface of the middle hepatic vein (MHV)/left hepatic vein (LHV) confluence towards the diaphragm exposing the confluence and the medial wall of the suprahepatic IVC.
- Display the upper surfaces of the MHV and LHV. Clear both veins of all tissue, exposing their junction with the IVC.
- The main trunk of the MHV usually joins the LHV, with a common trunk entering the IVC. The MHV may occasionally enter the IVC separately.

Cholecystectomy

- Perform a retrograde cholecystectomy.
- Incise the peritoneum overlying the CBD on the free edge of the lesser omentum extending up into Calot's triangle.
- Expose the cystic duct and cystic artery, ligating, and dividing them.
- The assistant retracts segment IV upwards with the right hand to expose the hilar plate and retracts the first part of the duodenum inferiorly with the left hand to expose the anterior surface of the hepatoduodenal ligament.
- Incise the hilar plate to expose the confluence of the right and left hepatic ducts.

Control inflow to the left lobe

- Carefully display the umbilical fissure.
- Elevate the ligamentum teres using the previously placed ligature.
- Divide the connecting bridge of liver tissue between segments III and IV using diathermy over a long curved artery forceps.
- The ligamentum teres can be seen entering the termination of the left portal vein (LPV) within the umbilical fissure.

- The triad of the LPV, LHA, and LHD enter at the base of the umbilical fissure to branch and supply segments II, III and IV.
- Open the peritoneum covering the left portion of the immediate subhilar area at the base of the umbilical ligament.
- Identify, ligate, and divide the LHA.
- A separate middle hepatic artery can sometimes be seen to the right of the LHA, entering the right side of the base of the umbilical fissure, and should be preserved if possible.
- The LPV is identified at the base of the umbilical fissure as it passes into the umbilical fissure.
- One or two major branches of the left portal triad arise just before these structures enter the umbilical fissure and pass postero-inferiorly to supply the caudate.
- Isolate the LPV, clamp, and divide it distal to the origin of the caudate lobe branches, at the base of the umbilical fissure.
- Identify the LHD above and behind the LPV, ligate and divide it. Under-run the LHD stump with 5/0 PDS.
- If the caudate lobe requires resection, the LPV, LHA, and LHD should be ligated close to the hilum to interrupt the supply to both the caudate and left liver.
- Inspect the gastrohepatic omentum for an accessory or replaced LHA arising from the left gastric artery. If present, ligate and divide it.
- **Technical variations:**
  - *en masse* extrahepatic left hepatic pedicle ligation with a mechanical stapler.
  - Intrahepatic division of the left hepatic pedicle.
  - Posterior intrahepatic Glissonian approach.

Isolate the middle and left hepatic veins
- Divide the gastrohepatic omentum using diathermy.
- Retract the left lobe to the right.
- Divide the ligamentum venosum close to the LHV.
- Develop a plane between the MHV and LHV.
- Pass a curved clamp between the LHV and IVC, emerging to the right of the MHV.
- Clamp, divide, and suture ligate the MHV and LHV separately using 4/0 prolene (or using a vascular stapler).

Parenchymal transection
- A line of demarcation should be visible from the mid-gallbladder fossa anteriorly to the left of the IVC posteriorly along the principle plane.
- Incise the capsule of the liver with diathermy 2mm lateral to the demarcation line created by pedicle division.
- Commence the parenchymal transection anteriorly through the middle of the base of the gallbladder fossa and proceed posteriorly.
- Continue anterior to the ligamentum venosum to separate the left liver from the anterior surface of the caudate lobe.
- Obtain haemostasis of the cut parenchymal surface.

Left lateral segmentectomy

Mobilize left lobe
- See Left hepatectomy 📖 p. 176.
- Cholecystectomy is not required.

Control inflow to left lobe
- See Left hepatectomy 📖 p. 176.
- Instead of isolating the LPV and LHA, individually isolate the portal pedicles to segments II and III, which should be clamped and ligated.
- Alternatively, isolate and divide the individual portal pedicles to segments II and III during parenchymal transection.

Isolate the left hepatic vein
- See Left hepatectomy 📖 p. 176.
- Pass a curved clamp between the LHV and IVC, emerging to the LEFT of the MHV, thereby isolating only the LHV.
- Clamp, divide, and suture ligate the LHV using 4/0 prolene (or using a vascular stapler).
- Alternatively, isolate and divide the LHV during parenchymal transection.

Parenchymal transection
- See Left hepatectomy 📖 p. 176.
- Transect the liver parenchyma in an anteroposterior direction just to the left of the ligamentum teres and falciform ligament, proceeding posteriorly and superiorly.
- Obtain haemostasis of the cut parenchymal surface. Place sutures into the capsule on either side of the cut surface.

Extended left hepatectomy

Definition
- Resection of segments [II, III] + IV + V + VIII ± I.
- Left hepatectomy extended to segment IV (+/– caudate lobe).
- High incidence of postoperative morbidity compared with left hepatectomy due to biliary complications and small-for-size.
- Plane of parenchymal transection is less clearly identified.

Mobilize left lobe
- See Left hepatectomy 📖 p. 176.
- IOUS may identify the presence of a large inferior RHV. If present, the main RHV may be sacrificed if necessary to achieve tumour clearance.

Limited mobilization of the right lobe
- Division of the ligamentous attachments of the right lobe allows palpation of segment VII for tumour and for later identification of the plane of parenchymal transection.
- Divide the right coronary ligament to expose the anterior surface of the suprahepatic IVC at the level of the major HV confluence.
- Divide the peritoneum over the right-hand side of the RHV to expose the right side of the suprahepatic IVC.
- The assistant lifts the liver upwards with the right hand to expose the hepatorenal ligament that is divided, exposing the lower border of the right lobe.
- The right lobe is retracted superomedially by the assistant's left hand to expose the right subphrenic space.
- Divide the inferior border of the triangular ligament.
- Divide the anterior layer of the right coronary ligament to meet the previous dissection lateral to the suprahepatic IVC.
- Divide the posterior layer of the right coronary ligament to the retrohepatic IVC.
- Divided the remaining inferior and superior leaves of the coronary ligament to expose the suprahepatic IVC.

Cholecystectomy
See Left hepatectomy 📖 p. 176.

Control inflow to the left lobe
- See Left hepatectomy 📖 p. 176.
- If resecting the caudate lobe the LPV, LHA, and LHD should be ligated close to the hilum to interrupt the supply to both the caudate and left lobe.

Isolate the middle and left hepatic veins
See Left hepatectomy 📖 p. 176.

Parenchymal transection

- The line of transection is horizontal along the obliterated ligamentum venosum, across the base of segment IV, curving inferolaterally to the right, extending parallel and anterior to the right scisura, lateral to galbladder bed and extending posteriorly to the anterior border of the RHV.
- Control inflow to segments V + VIII by clamping and dividing the right anterior sectoral pedicle.
- The right posterior pedicle is left intact.
- The posterior intrahepatic Glissonian approach can be performed to isolate and clamp the right anterior sectoral pedicle to assist in defining the line of demarcation for parenchymal transection.
- Alternatively, the right anterior sectoral vessels and bile ducts can be identified during parenchymal transection, and ligated/divided.
- Incise the capsule of the liver with diathermy 2mm lateral to the demarcation line created by pedicle division.
- Branches from the RHV are isolated, ligated, and divided.
- Once the right anterior sectoral pedicle has been identified, parenchymal transection proceeds along a plane anterior to the right posterior sectoral pedicle.
- The parenchymal transection just anterior to the ligamentum venosum separates the left liver from the anterior surface of the caudate.
- During parenchymal transection, the RHV must be preserved to its junction with the IVC (unless a large draining inferior RHV exists).
- Obtain haemostasis of the cut parenchymal surface.

Caudate lobe resection

Indications
- Isolated caudate resection for malignancy.
- Part of extended left or right hepatectomy for hilar cholangiocarcinoma. If performing preoperative right portal vein embolization (PVE) prior to extended right hepatectomy, the portal vein branch to segment IV should also be embolized.

Anatomical considerations
- Relations to surrounding structures: anterior-inferior (portal triad), posterior (IVC) and superior (IVC, MHV, and LHV).
- Divided into left and right portions separated by the ligamentum venosum. The left portion lies mainly to the left of the IVC and may extend to completely surround it.
- The gastrohepatic ligament inserts into the ligamentum venosum, separating the caudate lobe from the left lateral segment (II and III).
- Inferiorly, the caudate lobe passes between the portal vein and IVC, and superiorly under the LHV and MHV (anterolateral to the IVC) to fuse with segment VII.
- **Portal venous supply:** the smaller right portion received portal blood from the RPV or bifurcation of main PV. The larger left portion receives portal blood from the LPV
- **Arterial supply and biliary drainage:** right portion from right pedicle (RHA and RHD) or right posterior sectoral branches; left portion from left pedicle (LHA and LHD). Bile drains from caudate lobe via 3–5 ducts usually into LHD, but may be into both LHD and RHD, or occasionally to RHD.
- **Venous drainage:** directly into the IVC.

Resection technique
- Carefully display the umbilical fissure.
- Identify and ligate the caudate branches from the LPV and LHA.
- **Left approach:**
  - mobilize left lobe and retract to the right;
  - divide fibrous portion of caudate using diathermy;
  - lift the caudate lobe superolaterally;
  - individually ligate and divide caudate veins draining into the IVC.
- **Right approach:**
  - mobilize right lobe and retract to the left;
  - ligate and divide retrohepatic veins draining into IVC to expose major hepatic veins;
  - divide the parenchyma separating the caudate lobe from the IVC, segment IV and VII.
- Preserve the MHV if performing isolated caudate resection.

Right hepatectomy

General approach
- Bilateral subcostal +/– Mercedes extension or J-shaped incision.
- Exclude extrahepatic disease.
- Divide falciform ligament up to major hepatic veins.
- Perform IOUS to confirm site and size of lesion(s). Assess for additional lesions. Delineate arterial and venous anatomy.

Anatomical variation
- Segment IV may be supplied by a branch of the RHA. This should be preserved during hilar dissection.
- Segment IV bile duct frequently enters the RHD. To avoid injury, divide the RHD proximally in the liver parenchyma.
- Right posterior sectoral duct occasionally drains into the LHD. This is particularly important to recognize during left hepatectomy.
- Large inferior RHV may be present draining the posterior liver segments into the IVC. This must be identified, carefully dissected and divided between vascular clamps or stapler.

Mobilize the right lobe
- Bilateral subcostal or J-shaped incision.
- Adequate costal retraction.
- **Inflow occlusion:** intermittent Pringle manoeuvre.
- Divide and ligate the ligamentum teres (round ligament). Leave a long ligature on the divided ligamentum teres for later retraction.
- Divide the falciform ligament and separate from the upper anterior abdominal wall.
- The assistant's left-hand lowers the liver exposing the anterior layer of the right coronary ligament, which is divided until the anterior surface of the suprahepatic IVC is exposed at the level of the major hepatic vein (HV) confluence. The dissection should be performed close to the exposed liver substance.
- Divide the peritoneum over the right surface of the RHV towards the diaphragm exposing the right side of the suprahepatic IVC.
- The assistant lifts the liver upwards with the right hand exposing the hepatorenal ligament which is divided, exposing the lower border of the right lobe.
- The right lobe is retracted superomedially by the assistant's left hand to expose the right subphrenic space.
- Divide the inferior border of the triangular ligament.
- Divide the anterior layer of the right coronary ligament to meet the previous dissection lateral to the suprahepatic IVC.
- Divide the posterior layer of the right coronary ligament to the retrohepatic IVC.
- Divide the remaining inferior and superior leaves of the coronary ligament to expose the suprahepatic IVC.

- Divide the adhesions between the right lobe and retrohepatic space with gradual retraction of the liver medially, to expose the retrohepatic IVC and the adrenal gland, preserving the adrenal vein.
- Ligate any accessory adrenal veins entering the right lobe.

Control inflow to the right lobe

- Divide the peritoneal reflection along the free edge of the lesser omentum to expose the lateral side of the PV and CBD.
- Incise the peritoneum overlying the CBD on the free edge of the lesser omentum extending up into Calot's triangle.
- Perform a retrograde cholecystectomy.
- Expose the cystic duct and cystic artery, and ligate/divide them. Leave a tie on the CD for later retraction.
- The assistant retracts segment IV upwards with the right hand to expose the hilar plate and retracts the first part of the duodenum inferiorly with the left hand to expose the anterior surface of the hepatoduodenal ligament.
- Incise the hilar plate to expose the confluence of the RHD and LHD.
- Divide the peritoneum longitudinally on the right side of the porta hepatis, exposing, and encircling the PV. Further dissect cephalad to expose the LPV and RPV. Dissection is facilitated by gentle medial retraction of the CBD.
- Encircle the RPV with a vessel loop.
- Beware of the first posterior branch of the RPV, which comes off early and posteroinferiorly to supply the right portion of the caudate. Ligate and divide this branch if any difficulty is encountered.
- The right anterior and posterior sectoral PVs may be separate, and each may individually join the LPV confluence. In this case, the anterior and posterior sectoral PVs will need to be individually divided and secured.
- Identify the RHA in the lymphatic tissue anterior to the RPV. Ligate and divide the RHA to the right of the CBD.
- Divide the RPV between clamps and suture ligate, or use an endo-GIA vascular stapler.
- Divide the posterior hilar plate (may contain a small portal branch and bile duct, which should be ligated).
- Isolate, encircle, and divide the RHD with absorbable suture.
- Individually ligate, and divide the anterior and posterior sectoral ducts if entering the confluence separately.
- **Technical variations:**
  - *en masse* extrahepatic right hepatic pedicle ligation with a mechanical stapler;
  - intraparenchymal division of the right hepatic pedicle:
  - posterior intrahepatic Glissonian approach.

Complete mobilization of the right lobe

- The assistant retracts the liver superiorly to expose the infrahepatic IVC.
- The inferior RHV is ligated and divided if present (20% of patients).

- The hepatocaval ligament is divided exposing the right surface of the IVC.
- The spigelian veins are divided.
- With further cephalad dissection the inferior surface of the RHV is exposed.

Isolate the right hepatic vein

- The assistant retracts the liver inferiorly to expose the suprahepatic IVC.
- Divide the filamentous fibrous tissue between the RHV and MHV.
- Expose the left border of the RHV before it enters the suprahepatic IVC.
- The right lobe is retracted superomedially by the assistant to expose the IVC.
- Pass an atraumatic dissecting forceps around the RHV, and encircle it with a vessel loop.
- **Technical variation:** intraparenchymal division of the RHV during parenchymal transection.

Parenchymal transection

- Incise the capsule of the liver with diathermy 2mm lateral to the demarcation line created by pedicle division. Commence on the superior liver surface on the left edge of the RHV, along the interlobar fissure to the hilum, around the anterior border of segment I, cephalad along the posterior surface to the left edge of the RHV.
- Commence the parenchymal dissection anteriorly along the interlobar fissure with preservation of the MHV.
- On reaching the hilum, continue the dissection along the anterior border of segment I, towards the posterior and superior surfaces of the liver working cephalad.
- Divide the MHV branches to segments V + VIII.
- Once completely isolated, clamp the RHV, divide and suture ligate it, or use an endo-GIA vascular stapler.
- Obtain haemostasis of the cut parenchymal surface.

Extended right hepatectomy

Definition
- Resection of segments IV, V, VI, VII, VIII ± I.
- Right hepatectomy extended to segment IV.

Mobilize the right lobe
See Right hepatectomy 📖 p. 184.

Control inflow to the right lobe
- See Right hepatectomy 📖 p. 184.
- For extended right hepatectomy, it is essential to lower the hilar plater to enable visualization of the LHD. This also separates the LHD from the undersurface of segment IV.

Devascularization of segment IV
- Following inflow control to segments V, VI, VII, and VIII by extrahepatic dissection or pedicle control, the umbilical fissure of the liver should be carefully displayed.
- Elevate the ligamentum teres using the previously placed ligature.
- Divide the connecting bridge of liver tissue between segments III and IV using diathermy over a long curved artery forceps.
- The ligamentum teres can be seen entering the termination of the left portal vein (LPV) within the umbilical fissure.
- The triad of the LPV, LHA, and LHD enter at the base of the umbilical fissure to branch, and supply segments II, III, and IV.
- A separate middle hepatic artery can sometimes be seen running the right of the LHA, entering the right side of the base of the umbilical fissure.
- Close to the base of the umbilical fissure one or two major branches of the left portal triad passes posteroinferiorly to supply the caudate. Dividing these branches will devascularize the caudate lobe. Therefore, these branches need to be divided only when the caudate is being resected.
- Identify and divide the feedback vessels to segment IVa and IVb from the left portal triad within the umbilical fissure if the tumour margin is close. Division of these structures in the substance of the liver during parenchymal dissection to the right of the umbilical fissure can be performed in the absence of tumour adjacent to the umbilical fissure. Each vessel should be individually divided and suture ligated. This results in devacularization of segment IV.

Complete mobilization of the right lobe
See Right hepatectomy 📖 p. 184.

Isolate the right and middle hepatic veins

- The assistant retracts the liver inferiorly to expose the suprahepatic IVC.
- Divide the filamentous fibrous tissue between the RHV and MHV.
- Expose the left border of the RHV before it enters the suprahepatic IVC.
- The right lobe is retracted superomedially by the assistant to expose the IVC.
- Pass an atraumatic dissecting forceps around the RHV, and encircle it with a vessel loop.
- **Technical variation:** intraparenchymal division of the RHV during parenchymal transection.

Parenchymal transection

- After division of the portal pedicles to segments IV, V, VI, VII, VIII ± I, a line of demarcation should be visible.
- Incise the liver capsule using diathermy just to the right of the falciform ligament 2mm lateral to the demarcation line created by pedicle division.
- Parenchymal dissection begins anteriorly, proceeds posteriorly towards the umbilical fissure and extends posteriorly towards the IVC.
- On reaching the hilum, continue the dissection along the anterior border of segment I, towards the posterior and superior surfaces of the liver working cephalad.
- During the deeper, more posterior part of the parenchymal dissection the MHV is identified. To obtain tumour clearance, parenchymal transection is continued on the left side of the vein to reach its confluence with the IVC. The MHV can then be clamped, divided, and suture ligated, or divided with an Endo GIA stapler. Take care not to undermine or narrow the LHV.
- Once completely isolated, clamp the RHV, divide and suture ligate it, or use an endo-GIA vascular stapler.
- Minor branches should be secured and divided during parenchymal transection.
- Obtain haemostasis of the cut parenchymal surface.

Caudate lobe resection

- See Caudate resection 🕮 p. 182.
- For extended right hepatectomy the RPV and the portal branch to segment IV require embolization for optimal outcome.

Complications after liver resection

Early

Haemorrhage
- Significant postoperative bleeding in the first 24–48h may indicate technical error and requires immediate reoperation. Check clotting profile and correct abnormalities first.
- Delayed bleeding may present with acute fall in haemoglobin +/− hypovolaemic shock, and is usually related to intra-abdominal sepsis (+/− bile leak) leading to ruptured pseudo-aneurysm or disruption of venous staple/suture lines.
  - Stable patients should undergo CT angiography +/− embolization of bleeding pseudo-aneurysm and/or drainage of abscesses/bilomas. If a bile leak is confirmed, ERCP and stenting is indicated. Patients should receive broad-spectrum antibiotics and antifungal prophylaxis pending culture results.
  - Haemodynamically unstable patients should undergo immediate reoperation, with control of haemorrhage +/− abdominal packing. Once stabilized, further management should proceed as for stable patient.

Bile leak
- **Low volume:** likely source is cut surface, which usually resolves with conservative management (adequate drainage and IV antibiotics).
- **High volume:** indicates major duct leak, and requires ERCP, sphincterotomy, and stenting of the CBD to decompress the biliary tree and facilitate healing.

Collections
- Due to biloma, haematoma, or abscess.
- **Varied clinical presentation:** abdominal or shoulder tip pain, vomiting, fever, leukocytosis, overt sepsis/collapse.
- Abscesses should be aspirated and sent for culture.
- Bilomas should be treated by percutaneous drainage and IV antibiotics. Persistent, high volume bile drainage requires ERCP as above.

Small for size syndrome
- The optimum functioning liver mass should be 0.8–1% of body weight in the absence of parenchymal disease.
- Small for size syndrome (SFS) may develop after extended resections or standard resections if residual liver tissue is functionally impaired (e.g. segmental ischaemia, venous congestion). Morbidity and mortality occurs if resecting >60% estimated liver volume. Very high risk after resecting >75%.
- SFS may be prevented by preoperative right portal vein embolization 6 weeks before resection to allow left liver hypertrophy.
- Postoperatively, SFS presents with cholestasis, poor synthetic function, and sepsis.
- Presence of sepsis impairs liver regeneration, exacerbating the problem.

- Treatment is difficult and should include:
  - control of sepsis;
  - adequate biliary drainage;
  - treatment of associated organ failure.
- Recovery depends on adequate liver regeneration, which may take a prolonged time.
- Mortality is high.

Late

Biliary stricture
- Usually ischaemic in origin.
- Presents weeks or months postoperatively with obstructive jaundice, cholangitis or deranged liver function tests. Dilated ducts usually seen on US.
- Diagnosed by MRCP.
- Initial treatment is ERCP and balloon dilatation and/or stenting.
- Failed endoscopic treatment may require surgical revision (Roux-en-Y hepatico-jejunostomy).

Portal vein stenosis
Technical complication or may be secondary to stretching of the vein with liver growth. Leads to portal hypertension (ascites, varices, encephalopathy). Treated by transhepatic portal vein stenting.

Venous outflow occlusion
- Rare.
- May be due to torsion of liver remnant (due to failure to anchor liver) or undermining of LHV.

Liver trauma

O. Tucker

Mechanism of injury

Mode of injury

Blunt
- The main cause of death after major blunt abdominal trauma (mortality rate 10–31%).
- Mortality related to AAST grading of liver injury (see Table 8.1).
- Injury may be due to direct blow, shearing, or rotational force, or deceleration injury.
- Associated other injuries common.

See Fig. 8.1.

Penetrating
- Isolated penetrating injury becoming more prevalent in UK.
- Stab wound more common than gunshot wound.
- Liver at risk after any penetrating thoracoabdominal or abdominal injury.

Table 8.1 AAST grading of liver injury

	Haematoma	Laceration
I	Subcapsular – <10% surface area	<1cm deep
II	Subcapsular – 10–50% surface area Parenchymal – <10cm diameter	1–3cm deep <10cm long
III	Subcapsular – >50% surface area, expanding or ruptured Parenchymal – >10cm or expanding	>3cm deep
IV		Parenchymal disruption 25–75% one lobe
V		Parenchymal disruption >75% one lobe Hepatic vein or retrohepatic caval injury
VI		Hepatic avulsion

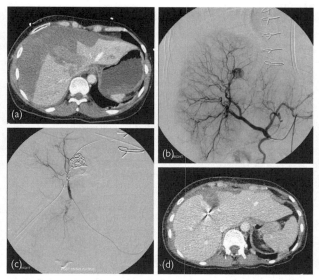

Fig. 8.1 Blunt liver trauma. (a) CT scan of a patient who sustained a severe blunt injury to the liver, with deep laceration extending into the hilum. The patient was initially haemodynamically stable and managed non-operatively, but later required radiographic embolization due to arterial bleeding (b,c). The CT appearances after 4 weeks are shown in (d).

Non-operative management

Initial assessment and resuscitation

- **ATLS principles:** airway/cervical spine control, respiratory support/high flow oxygen, intravenous access, fluid resuscitation, and haemorrhage control. Exclude other injuries (log roll the patient).
- Exclude tension pneumothorax, massive haemothorax (examine chest), or cardiac tamponade (injury medial to nipples +/– echocardiogram or fast scan) as cause for persistent hypotension in patient with penetrating thoracoabdominal injury.
- Apply direct pressure to bleeding abdominal wall vessels.
- If suspected arterial injury in shocked patient → 'hypotensive resuscitation' aiming to maintain perfusion to brain (conscious patient) and emergency transfer to theatre for surgical control of haemorrhage.
- **Indications for immediate laparotomy:** unstable/hypotensive despite resuscitation, bowel evisceration, peritonitis, and all abdominal gunshot wounds.
- In stable patient, probe wound with sterile microbiology swab. If peritoneal breach obvious, consider laparotomy, rather than CT.
- If no peritoneal breach evident and patient stable → CT with IV contrast.

Stable patient with blunt liver injury

- **Non-operative management (NOM):** successful in 90% of patients with liver injuries who are haemodynamically stable, irrespective of AAST grade of injury. Higher grade injuries more likely to need intervention (angiographic embolization or surgery), and have a higher mortality.
- **Contraindications to NOM of blunt liver injury:** hypotension, peritonitis, suspected other injuries (e.g. bowel perforation on CT), lack of availability of HDU/ITU care.
- **NOM involves:**
  - invasive BP/CVP monitoring in HDU/ITU setting;
  - frequent clinical re-evaluation by experienced surgeon;
  - serial CT scan after 5–7 days (to assess evolution of injury, exclude pseudoaneurysm or biloma/bile leak);
  - percutaneous drainage of bilomas.
- **Indications for selective hepatic angiography:** arterial bleeding on CT angiography, significant/ongoing transfusion requirement. Selective embolization of a bleeding point may be used as a primary intervention, pre-operatively in a patient who requires abdominal decompression, or post-operatively in a patient with ongoing bleeding after perihepatic packing.
- **Indications for surgery:** haemodynamic instability, massive haemoperitoneum causing abdominal compartment syndrome (intra-abdominal pressure >20mmHg in the presence of respiratory or renal dysfunction), failed angiographic haemostasis, or biliary peritonitis due to uncontained bile leak.
- In general, timing of intervention should be dictated primarily by clinical course, rather than CT findings.

- **Indication for ERCP and biliary stent:** if persistent bile leak after drainage. ERCP may confirm site of leak, and allows insertion of a CBD stent to facilitate resolution of small leaks(Fig. 8.2).

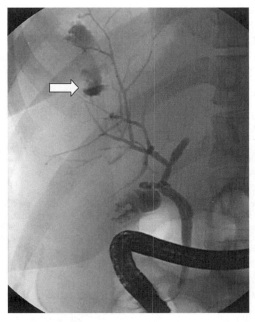

Fig. 8.2 Bile leak after liver trauma. ERCP in a patient after blunt liver trauma, which demonstrates a peripheral bile leak (arrowed) and incidental gallstones. A plastic stent was inserted into the common bile duct and the leak subsequently resolved.

Surgical management

- **Pre-requisites:**
  - experienced surgeon and anaesthetist;
  - available blood products (including FFP and platelets);
  - available ITU bed;
  - interventional radiology support.
- Management of severe liver trauma in tertiary HPB centres associated with reduced morbidity and mortality. However, aggressive resusciatation +/– perihepatic packing at the referring hospital are essential.
- Patients that require surgical intervention have a higher Injury Severity Score, lower Glasgow Coma Score (GCS), lower BP, higher fluid/blood requirement, and increased liver-related mortality.
- Incision: midline or bilateral subcostal (+/– vertical extension).
- Four-quadrant packing.
- Allow patient to be fluid resuscitated.
- Assess nature/extent of liver injury.
- Exclude other injuries.
- Perform perihepatic packing (see Surgical management, Perihepatic packing 🕮 p. 198). If bleeding controlled, perform 'damage control', close abdomen, and return to theatre in 36–72h. If bleeding NOT controlled by packing, options include: hepatic in-flow occlusion (Pringle manoeuvre) or aortic cross-clamping. If still bleeding after packing *and* in-flow occlusion, suggests HV or retrohepatic IVC injury (high mortality).
- Other surgical options include selective HA ligation, resectional debridement, anatomical resection, total hepatectomy + emergency liver transplantation. These options have a mortality >50% and are rarely required. They should not be performed outside a tertiary HPB centre. If RHA ligated, cholecystectomy should be performed.
- **Retrohepatic caval injury:** call perfusionist. Set up venovenous bypass (femoral vein to axillary or internal jugular vein). Perform total vascular isolation (in-flow occlusion and clamping of supra- and infra-hepatic IVC).

Perihepatic packing

- Packing is the key to a successful outcome.
- Simple, effective technique to achieve haemostasis.
- Reduces blood transfusion requirements.
- Does not require specialist instruments or tertiary facilities.
- Reduces infection and mortality.
- Divide the falciform ligament only. No further mobilization should be necessary.
- Place packs to compress injured liver from side to side (Fig. 8.3).
- To prevent abdominal compartment syndrome close the skin only, or suture silastic mesh/Bogota bag to fascia.
- Administer broad spectrum antibiotics and antifungals.

❶ Don't pack into fractures.

❶ Don't over-pack.

❶ Don't lift the liver up (risk of air embolism).

❶ Avoid compressing the IVC and renal vein with subhepatic packs.

❶ Damage control laparotomy with perihepatic packing followed by angio-embolization confers an increased survival benefit compared with early laparotomy with definite haemostasis.

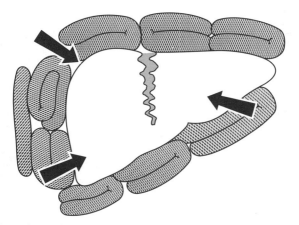

Fig. 8.3 Liver packing.

- Remove packs at 36–72h. Allows correction of hypothermia, acidosis and coagulopathy, and allows clot to mature. Risk of rebleeding after pack removal.

Total hepatectomy and liver transplantation
- **Indications:** uncontrollable liver haemorrhage, liver failure, severe *post-reperfusion injury* (see Anaesthetic considerations, Reperfusion syndrome).
- Should only be performed in association with advice from a transplant centre.
- Perform hepatectomy and temporary portocaval shunt.
- Transfer to ITU and list patient for super-urgent transplant.

Postoperative care following liver injury
- Nasogastric tube feeding.
- Antibiotics.
- Invasive monitoring and/or organ support as indicated.
- Routine CT angiogram after 7–10 days to exclude hepatic artery pseudoaneurysm.

- Frequent USS to assess for bile collection (treat by percutaneous drainage and ERCP/stent).

Restrict activity for 6 weeks (not evidence-based).

Complications after liver injury

- Usually develop after 10–14 days. Preceded by low grade persistent fever.
- Sepsis.
- Bile leak.
- Biliary stricture.
- Pseudoaneurysm.
- Haemobilia.
- Arterioportal fistula.

Liver tumour ablation

R. Sutcliffe

Transarterial chemo-embolization

Indications
- Unresectable HCC.
- Disease control in HCC patients suitable for liver transplant.

Contra-indications
- Portal vein thrombosis (relative).
- Impaired renal function (relative).
- Decompensated liver disease (ascites, jaundice, or encephalopathy).

Technique
- Primary liver tumours derive their blood supply principally from the hepatic artery rather than portal vein.
- TACE involves delivery of chemotherapeutic agents (e.g. doxorubicin, cisplatin, mitomycin, 5-fluorouracil) directly into a tumour via a cannula positioned in the hepatic artery or its branches. This reduces systemic toxicity of these agents. Subsequent embolization renders the tumour ischaemic.

Results
- TACE provides symptomatic relief in significant proportion.
- Some evidence of improved survival in patients with HCC and colorectal liver metastases (CLM) (Llovet et al., 2002; Lo et al., 2002).
- Arterial embolization alone without chemotherapeutic agents may be as effective as TACE for unresectable HCC. Chemotherapy component important in CLM.

Complications
- Post-embolization syndrome (see Box 9.1).
- Sepsis (e.g. cholecystitis, liver abscess).
- Gastrointestinal bleeding.
- Liver failure.
- Renal failure (due to iodinated radiocontrast medium).

Box 9.1 Post-embolization syndrome

- Common after all ablation techniques.
- Characterized by abdominal pain, fever, malaise, and transient derangement of liver function.
- Treatment is supportive.
- Exclude liver failure.

Further information

Llovet, J.M., Real, M.I., Montaña, X., Planas, R., Coll, S., Aponte, J., Ayuso, C., Sala, M., Muchart, J., Solà, R., Rodés, J., Bruix, J., and the Barcelona Liver Cancer Group. (2002) Arterial embolisation or chemoembolisation versus symptomatic treatment in patients with unresectable hepatocellular carcinoma: a randomised controlled trial. *Lancet* **359**(9319), 1734–9.

Lo, C.M., Ngan, H., Tso, W.K., Liu, C.L., Lam, C.M., Poon, R.T., Fan, S.T., & Wong, J. ((2002) Randomized controlled trial of transarterial lipiodol chemoembolization for unresectable hepatocellular carcinoma. *Hepatology* **35**, 1164–71.

Percutaneous ethanol injection

Indications
Unresectable HCC less than 3cm.

Contra-indications
None.

Technique
- Pure ethanol is injected directly into the tumour, causing necrosis by protein denaturation and vascular thrombosis.
- Spread of ethanol to normal liver is limited by the presence of a capsule.

Results
- Tumour recurrence is common.
- Often requires repeat injections.

Complications
- Uncommon.
- Post-embolization syndrome.

Radiofrequency thermal ablation

Indications
- Unresectable HCC (including large tumours).
- Colorectal liver metastases.
- Unresectable neuroendocrine liver metastases.

Contra-indications
Presence of extrahepatic disease (except neuroendocrine tumours).

Technique
- RFA may be administered percutaneously (using US or CT guidance) or during open/laparoscopic surgery. Requires sedation or general anaesthesia.
- Radiofrequency energy (via alternating current) induces ionic agitation and heat in surrounding tissues (up to 100°), leading to tumour necrosis (1.5cm radius).
- For large tumours (up to 8cm), need multiple placement and deployment of electrode in overlapping zones. Aim to destroy tumour plus 1cm margin of normal liver.
- During open surgery, hepatic artery inflow occlusion minimizes cooling effect of circulating blood, thereby increasing therapeutic effect.

Results
- RFA produces a larger area of ablation than other techniques and may be associated with improved survival (Cochrane review, 2002).
- Useful for palliation of multiple neuroendocrine liver metastases.
- Survival similar to PEI, but less recurrence with RFA in randomized controlled trials.

Complications
- Post-embolization syndrome.
- Heat injury to adjacent structures.
- Liver failure.

Further information
Galandi, D., & Antes, G. (2004) Radiofrequency thermal ablation versus other interventions for hepatocellular carcinoma. *Cochrane Database Syst Rev* **2**, CD003046.

Yttrium microspheres

Indications
- Unresectable primary and metastatic liver tumours.
- Relatively new technique. Benefit vs. other ablation techniques is unknown.

Contra-indications
- Significant intrahepatic shunt (microspheres pass into pulmonary circulation and can cause radiation pneumonitis).
- Radiation gastritis due to microspheres passing into gastric branches of CHA.

Technique
- Radioactive yttrium-90 microspheres (20–60μm diameter) are injected into the hepatic artery (via transfemoral artery catheter) and delivered to the liver tumour.
- Side branches (e.g. to stomach) should be embolized before injection.
- Microspheres emit β-radiation to tumour, sparing normal liver.
- PET scans are better than CT in evaluating response to therapy and allow estimation of tumour bulk.

Results
- Encouraging early results in hepatocellular carcinoma, colorectal, and neuroendocrine liver metastases in terms of radiological response.
- There may be a potential synergistic effect with chemotherapy for colorectal metastases.
- Results of RCTs and long-term follow-up data are awaited.

Complications
- Post-embolization syndrome common.
- Radiation pneumonitis (if significant intrahepatic shunt).
- Radiation hepatitis (liver decompensation).
- Peptic ulceration (radiation gastritis).
- Late cholangiopathy.

Biliary diseases

R. Sutcliffe, N. Battula, & T. Pirani

Bile duct obstruction

Aetiology

Bile duct obstruction may be *complete, incomplete,* or *segmental.* The type of obstruction differs in different disease processes (see Table 10.1).

Pathophysiology

Local effects (see Table 10.2)

- Bile duct obstruction results in elevated CBD pressure, which inhibits bile production. Proximal dilatation of the biliary tree is common in bile duct obstruction, but may be absent with chronic inflammation, fibrosis or cirrhosis. Presence of severe pain suggests CBD obstruction may due to a stone, rather than a neoplasm.
- The histological effects of bile duct obstruction are similar to those seen in *intrahepatic cholestasis*. Bile duct proliferation and portal tract inflammation (acute cholangiolitis). Excess bile salts are toxic to hepatocytes and may lead to cell necrosis by an unknown mechanism. In cases of prolonged bile duct obstruction (weeks-months), periportal fibrosis may develop, eventually leading to *portal hypertension. Secondary biliary cirrhosis* occurs late if the obstruction is not relieved. Patients with incomplete obstruction (e.g. iatrogenic CBD stricture) may not become jaundiced, but instead present late with portal hypertension. Recovery of hepatocyte function may take up to 6 weeks following relief of bile duct obstruction. Fibrotic changes (before the onset of cirrhosis) may also be reversed to some extent by effective biliary drainage.
- Bile duct obstruction predisposes to bacterial infection (*ascending cholangitis*) due to the presence of bile stasis (particularly in the presence of CBD stones) and raised CBD pressure. Gram-negative organisms, such as *Escherichia coli* and *Enterococcus* spp. are the commonest cause of cholangitis, and in the presence of bile stasis may lead to *primary CBD stones.*

Systemic effects (see Table 10.2)

Patients with obstructive jaundice are at risk of developing systemic inflammatory response (SIRS) and multiple organ dysfunction (MODS). The mechanism is incompletely understood, but there is evidence that this may be secondary to endotoxinaemia. Lack of bile salts in the intestine alters small bowel microflora, which is associated with increased intestinal permeability and predisposes to bacterial translocation. In addition, bile salts inhibit the hepatic reticulo-endothelial system leading to reduced clearance of endotoxin from the portal circulation.

Table 10.1 Causes of bile duct obstruction

Type I (complete)	Carcinoma of the head of pancreas
	Cholangiocarcinoma
	Intrahepatic tumours (primary & secondary)
	Ligation/division of CBD
Type II (intermittent)	CBD stones
	Ampullary tumour
	Bile duct papilloma
	Duodenal diverticulum
	Choledochal cyst
	Biliary parasitic infection
	Haemobilia
Type III (incomplete)	CBD stricture (e.g. iatrogenic, PSC, radiation)
	Bilio-enteric anastomotic stricture
	Chronic pancreatitis
	Sphincter of Oddi dysfunction
Type IV (segmental)	Trauma
	Hepatic duct stones
	PSC
	Cholangiocarcinoma

Table 10.2 Complications of bile duct obstruction

Local	Systemic
Hepatocyte necrosis	Systemic inflammatory Response (SIRS)
Periportal fibrosis	Multiple organ dysfunction
Portal hypertension	
Secondary biliary cirrhosis	
Ascending cholangitis	
Primary CBD stones	
Multiple organ dysfunction	

Gallstones

Pathology
- Prevalence 10–20%.
- More common in women (F:M = 2:1) and increasing age.
- Risk factors for gallstone formation are shown in Table 10.3.

Cholesterol stones
- Account for 75% of gallstones in the West.
- In patients in whom bile is supersaturated with cholesterol, precipitation/stone formation depends on balance of factors (e.g. mucin glycoproteins, lipoproteins, gallbladder stasis, genetic predisposition).

Black pigment stones
- Account for 25% of stones in the West.
- Excess unconjugated bilirubin polymerizes and/or precipitates with Ca^{2+} (haemolysis, liver disease).

Brown pigment stones
- Form predominantly within the ducts.
- Associated with biliary infection.
- Composed of Ca^{2+} bilirubinate and small amounts of cholesterol bound to organic material.

Table 10.3 Risk factors for gallstone formation

Cholesterol stones	Pigment stones
Genetic	Haemolytic disease
Cystic fibrosis	Biliary infections (bacterial, parasitic)
Age	Cirrhosis
Female sex	Crohn's disease
Obesity	
Diabetes mellitus	

Clinical spectrum of gallstones

Epidemiology
- 50,000 cholecystectomies performed each year in the UK.
- More than 100,000 hospital admissions per year with symptomatic gallstones.

Asymptomatic gallstones
- 10–20% of the population develop gallstones.
- The majority of patients are asymptomatic (85%).
- 1–4% of patients with gallstones will develop symptoms per year.
- It is not possible to predict which subgroup of patients will become symptomatic and, therefore, cholecystectomy cannot be recommended routinely in asymptomatic patients, with the exception of patients with sickle cell anaemia or a calcified gallbladder (13–22% risk of carcinoma).

Biliary colic
- Classical symptom associated with gallstones causing obstruction (Hartmann's pouch, cystic duct, common bile duct).
- Characterized by severe, sharp RUQ pain radiating to back/ shoulder tip.
- Not always 'colicky' (may be constant).
- Usually episodic and often associated with fatty meals.
- Diagnose by typical history combined with RUQ tenderness (Murphy's sign) and presence of gallstones on ultrasound.
- Exclude other causes of RUQ/epigastric pain (e.g. peptic ulcer, ruptured AAA, pancreatitis, hepatitis) by careful history, examination and investigations.
- Distinguish biliary colic from *acute calculous cholecystitis*, *acute pancreatitis*, *obstructive jaundice*, *ascending cholangitis* (see Table 10.4) by:
  - nature and characteristics of pain;
  - presence/absence of jaundice;
  - presence/absence of fever (and leukocytosis).
- Treatment is symptomatic using strong analgesics (e.g. NSAIDs, opiates). Admission to hospital may be required in severe cases. Elective laparoscopic cholecystectomy is indicated if symptoms are severe and/or persistent.

Acute cholecystitis
See Acute cholecystitis 📖 p. 214.

Obstructive jaundice
See Obstructive jaundice 📖 p. 216.

Acute pancreatitis
See Acute pancreatitis 📖 p. 240.

Table 10.4 Clinical spectrum of gallstones

	Pain	Vomiting	Jaundice	Fever
Biliary colic	Colicky RUQ	+/–	–	–
Acute cholecystitis	RUQ → shoulder	+	–	+
Acute pancreatitis	Epigastric → back	+++	+/–	+/–
Common bile duct stone	RUQ → shoulder	+	++	–
Ascending cholangitis	RUQ → shoulder	+	++	++

Acute cholecystitis

Pathology

Acute calculous cholecystitis
- Gallstone impacted in Hartmanns pouch.
- Chemical cholecystitis progresses to bacterial cholecystitis in 30% (*E. coli*, *Klebsiella* spp., *Strep. faecalis*).
- Mucocoele/empyema may develop if gallbladder obstructed.
- Gangrene +/− perforation occurs especially in the elderly, HIV patients, diabetics and in *acute acalculous cholecystitis*.

Acute acalculous cholecystitis
- Occurs in critically ill patients (trauma, diabetes, burns, sepsis, post-operatively).
- Gangrene occurs in up to 60% of cases and mortality is high (40%).

Clinical features

Symptoms
- RUQ pain radiating to back/shoulder.
- Nausea and vomiting are common.

Signs
- Fever and marked tenderness in the RUQ (positive Murphy's sign).
- A palpable tender gallbladder suggests a mucocoele or empyema.

Differential diagnosis
- Perforated peptic ulcer.
- Pancreatitis.
- Appendicitis.
- Hepatitis.

Investigations

- Neutrophil leukocytosis is common.
- Only 10% of gallstones are visible on plain abdominal X-ray.
- Ultrasonography within 24–48h looking for calculi, sludge, thickened gallbladder wall, and pericholecystic oedema.
- HIDA scan may be useful if US not diagnostic.
- *Acute acalculous cholecystitis* can be diagnosed by CCK cholescintigraphy with 98% sensitivity.

Management

- Patients should be kept NBM and given IV fluids.
- Intravenous cephalosporin or ciprofloxacin should be administered (e.g. IV cefuroxime 750mg tds *or* ciprofloxacin 200–400mg bd).
- Strong analgesia is usually required (e.g. combination of regular IV paracetamol 1g qds *plus* PO diclofenac 50mg tds *plus* IV morphine 5-10mg prn).
- Patients should be reviewed regularly to look for signs of clinical deterioration including peritonitis (suggesting gallbladder perforation or missed peptic ulcer), septic shock, and jaundice (suggesting ascending cholangitis).

- Presence of peritonitis mandates urgent surgery (laparoscopic or open cholecystectomy via Kocher's incision).
- If the patient's condition responds to conservative treatment, they should undergo laparoscopic cholecystectomy *either* during the same admission *or* within 6–8 weeks.

Complications of cholecystitis

Gallbladder perforation

- Cholecystitis may progress to gangrene followed by perforation.
- Patients present with sepsis and peritonitis.
- Treat by resuscitation followed by urgent open cholecystectomy.

Empyema

- Clinical features similar to cholecystitis, except patients are more unwell with high fever and tender, palpable GB.
- Treat as for cholecystitis plus consider US-guided aspiration of pus, followed by emergency cholecystectomy.
- Differential diagnosis is a mucocoele: patients have a tender palpable GB, but no signs of sepsis.

Gallbladder carcinoma

- Rare complication of chronic cholecystitis.
- Patients usually present late with local and/or distant spread.
- In patients with localized disease, cholecystectomy is indicated.

Gallstone ileus

- Rare complication of cholecystitis in which a fistula develops between the gallbladder fundus and the duodenal cap (cholecystoduodenal fistula). Usually occurs in the elderly.
- This allows passage of a large gallstone into the intestine, causing small bowel obstruction by impaction at the ileocaecal valve.
- Gas in the biliary tree in the presence of features of small bowel obstruction on a plain abdominal X-ray is diagnostic.
- Treat by urgent laparotomy. The gallstone is retrieved via a longitudinal enterotomy (closed transversely to prevent stricture formation) in the distal ileum. Presence of gangrene +/− perforation may require small bowel resection +/− primary anastomosis. Cholecystectomy is contra-indicated in patients with a cholecystoduodenal fistula.

Obstructive jaundice

- A partially obstructed CBD may lead to a minor elevation of serum alkaline phosphatase.
- Complete obstruction presents with abdominal pain and features of obstructive jaundice (including pale stools and dark urine).
- Take a full history and perform physical examination.
- If the patient looks unwell and is pyrexial, consider *ascending cholangitis*.
- Look for signs of other causes of jaundice (e.g. risk factors for hepatitis, signs of chronic liver disease).
- Routine blood tests (FBC, U&E, LFTs, amylase, clotting profile, G&S).
- Ultrasound will show gallstones in GB and may demonstrate dilated intra- and extrahepatic bile ducts, but is insensitive for detecting CBD stones.
- If clinical features and US findings consistent with obstructive jaundice, check clotting and arrange an ERCP (see Fig. 10.1).
- If low index of suspicion (e.g. 'hepatitic' LFTs, no gallstones, and/or normal CBD diameter on US), investigate for other causes of jaundice (hepatitis screen: viral serology, autoantibodies, immunoglobulin).
- If still considering bile duct obstruction, arrange MRCP or endoscopic US to look for pancreatic pathology and CBD stones. Proceed to ERCP if positive MRCP. If clinical features indicate possible malignancy, arrange CT with contrast and check tumour markers (CA-19.9, CEA).

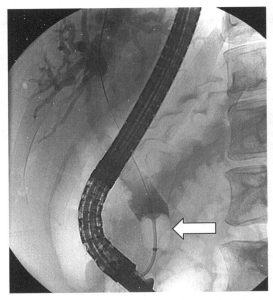

Fig. 10.1 Common bile duct stone. ERCP demonstrating stone in distal end of common bile duct.

Common bile duct stones

Pathology
- Majority of common bile duct (CBD) stones are *secondary*, originating in the gallbladder.
- Primary CBD stones are rare and diagnosed by the presence of stones/sludge in CBD in the absence of long cystic duct remnant or biliary stricture in a patient who has been asymptomatic for >2 years after cholecystectomy.
- Common in patients with choledochal anomalies.

Clinical features
- CBD stones may be asymptomatic or present with:
  - biliary colic;
  - acute pancreatitis;
  - obstructive jaundice;
  - ascending cholangitis.
- CBD stones should be excluded in all patients prior to laparoscopic cholecystectomy, i.e. no recent history of jaundice, normal liver function tests, and no ultrasonographic evidence of CBD dilatation (normal CBD less than 9mm).
- If CBD stones are suspected, MRCP or endoscopic US should be performed, proceeding to ERCP and stone removal if CBD stone detected.
- 10–15% of patients undergoing cholecystectomy will have unsuspected stones in the CBD requiring further intervention and it has been advocated that intraoperative cholangiography should be performed routinely in all patients.
- Presence of Charcot's triad (fever, pain, and jaundice) indicates ascending cholangitis, which may be associated with signs of septic shock and confusion (Reynold's pentad) in severe cases.

Management
- In patients with ascending cholangitis, prompt resuscitation with IV fluids, IV antibiotics, and close monitoring in HDU or ITU are essential. Supportive treatment of organ failure may be necessary. ERCP should be performed on the next available list.
- ERCP and stone removal is the treatment of choice for CBD stones. Sphincterotomy is performed and stones extracted using a balloon-tipped catheter or wire basket +/– stent placement if residual stones.
- Refractory stones may be cleared by lithotripsy (mechanical, electrohydraulic or laser).
- In patients with proven CBD stones, surgical exploration of CBD is indicated if:
  - ERCP not possible, unavailable or unsuccessful;
  - stone palpated during open cholecystectomy;
  - stone detected by intraoperative cholangiography during laparoscopic cholecystectomy.

Common bile duct exploration

Transcystic approach
- Insert choledochoscope into cystic duct via a 5mm port.
- Extract stones using a Nitinol basket through the working channel.

Choledochotomy
- Dissect peritoneum from anterior aspect of CBD.
- Aspirate bile to confirm its location.
- Perform longitudinal choledochotomy using a size 15 blade and Pott's scissors.
- Insert choledochoscope and remove CBD stone as above.
- If the CBD is cleared, close the choledochotomy primarily using interrupted 5/0 PDS. Leave a drain in the subhepatic space.
- If the CBD has not been cleared, close the choledochotomy over a T-tube (each limb cut to 1cm using fine tenotomy scissors), using 5/0 PDS, taking care not to occlude or kink the T-tube (Fig. 10.2).
- Bring the end of the T-tube out through a separate skin incision without tension and securely suture to the skin using 2/0 silk.
- If the T-tube falls out in the early postoperative period, the patient should be returned to theatre, the abdomen washed out, and the T-tube re-inserted.

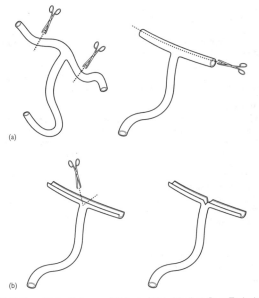

(a)

(b)

Fig. 10.2 Cutting a T-tube. Cut arms of T-tube to fit into bile duct. Open T-tube by cutting across as shown in (a). Create V-shaped nick at junction (b), to facilitate removal.

Intrahepatic stones

Pathology

- Rare in Western counties, prevalent in East Asia.
- Intrahepatic stones are either cholesterol or mixed, and are associated with biliary infection (*E. coli*, *Clostridium* spp., *Bacteroides* spp.).
- Bacterial e-glucuronidase causes hydrolysis of conjugated bilirubin, leading to precipitation of Ca^{2+} bilirubinate salts in the biliary tree.
- Left lobe affected more than right lobe possibly due to bile stasis.

Clinical features

Symptoms
- Right upper quadrant pain.
- Fever and jaundice develop in up to 30%.

Investigations
- US detects stones +/– duct dilatation.
- CT and MRCP is needed to define anatomical location of stones and look for abscesses and signs of portal hypertension due to biliary cirrhosis.
- For right-sided or bilateral stones, visualize the ducts by percutaneous transhepatic cholangiography, or cholangioscopy.

Management

- Urgent percutaneous transhepatic biliary drainage if obstruction or cholangitis. Try to remove intrahepatic stones using percutaneous transhepatic cholangioscopy. The role of stents is unclear.
- Supportive treatment for cholangitis: IV fluids, IV antibiotics, organ support (HDU or ITU).
- Consider hepatic resection if:
  - atrophic liver segment;
  - multiple intrahepatic strictures;
  - cystic dilatation of peripheral ducts.
- If stricture is present at RHD, LHD, or hepatic confluence, consider Roux-en-Y hepatico-jejunostomy.

Gallbladder carcinoma

Epidemiology
- Rare malignancy.
- Highest incidence in Chile, north eastern Europe, Israel, and South America.
- F > M.
- Increased incidence with age.

Aetiology
- Frequently associated with gallstones and cholecystitis.
- 10–25% of porcelain gallbladders are associated with cancer.
- Chemicals like methyldopa, isoniazid, oral contraceptives, and occupational exposure in rubber industry have been implicated in carcinogenesis.
- Associated with common channel between pancreatic and bile ducts.

Pathology
- Usually arises in fundus or neck.
- Adenocarcinoma in 90%. Less common types are papillary, mucinous, and squamous cell carcinoma.
- Spreads early via local invasion, lymphatic and haematogenous routes.

Clinical features
- Right upper quadrant pain.
- Mass.
- Weight loss.
- Jaundice due to biliary obstruction or large volume liver metastases.
- Cholecystitis.

Investigations
- LFTs.
- CA 19.9.
- US.
- CT to stage disease.
- MRI/MRCP if considering curative resection.
- ERCP if jaundiced.

Management
- Determined by radiological TNM staging (see Table 10.5).
- May be diagnosed on histological analysis after cholecystectomy.
- Majority of patients have unresectable disease and/or metastases at the time of diagnosis.

T1 tumours
Cholecystectomy. 5-year survival 85–100%.

T2 tumours
Gallbladder bed resection. 5-year survival 60–70% (Fig. 10.4).

T3 tumours
- Extended right hepatectomy +/− excision of the extrahepatic biliary tree if the cystic duct margin is involved (frozen section). Preoperative right portal vein embolization if small future liver remnant. 5-year survival 20%.
- There is no proven role for adjuvant chemotherapy or radiotherapy.
- Potential survival benefit with gemcitabine or cisplatin-based regimens.

Unresectable tumours (T4 or N1 or M1 disease)
- Metallic biliary stenting.
- Palliative chemotherapy if good performance status (Fig 10.5).

Table 10.5 TNM staging of gallbladder carcinoma

T1	Carcinoma *in situ*
T2	Invades muscle layer
T3	Invades serosa, or direct invasion into adjacent liver and/or involves one adjacent organ
T4	Invades portal vein, hepatic artery or two or more adjacent organs
N0	No regional lymph node metastases
N1	Regional lymph node metastase
M0	No distant metastases
M1	Distant metastases

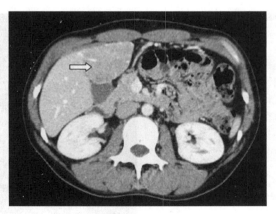

Fig. 10.3 Focal nodular hyperplasia.

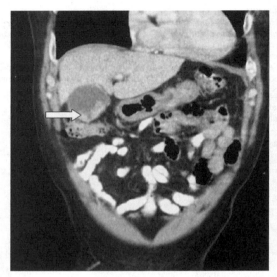

Fig. 10.4 Gallbladder cancer. Resectable gallbladder cancer.

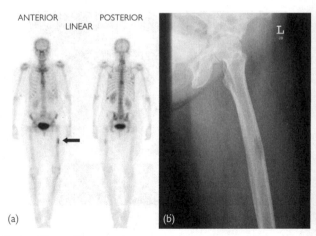

Fig. 10.5 X-ray and bone scan of a patient with a metastasis in the left femur after previous liver resection for gallbladder cancer.

Laparoscopic cholecystectomy

Indications
- Symptomatic gallstones.
- Gallbladder polyp.
- Acalculous cholecystitis.
- Perforated gallbladder.

Relative contra-indications
- Significant comorbidity.
- Previous upper abdominal surgery.
- Portal hypertension and varices.
- Pregnancy.

Preoperative work-up
- Check FBC, U&E, and clotting profile.
- Confirm diagnosis by clinical features and positive US.
- **Check LFTS:** if deranged, arrange MRCP to evaluate for common bile duct stones. ERCP and stone retrieval if MRCP shows CBD stone.
- **Consent:** document specific risks – conversion to open operation (5%), bleeding, bile duct injury, bile leak, bowel injury, pain, wound infection.
- Position the anaesthetized patient supine on the operating table, prepare the skin of the anterior abdominal wall (including costal margins) with aqueous betadine solution.

Creating the pneumoperitoneum
- The open (Hasson) technique for establishing a pneumoperitoneum is preferred over Veress needle insufflation (Fig. 10.6).
- Make a 1.5cm long vertical or transverse periumbilical incision (above or below the umbilicus).
- Extend the incision through subcutaneous tissue.
- Elevate the umbilicus using Allis forceps and incise the linea alba.
- Penetrate the parietal peritoneum with closed McIndoe scissors.
- Insert a 10mm port using a blunt trocar and connect the CO_2 supply to it on high flow.
- Set the maximum pressure to 12mmHg. Ensure that there is no resistance to the flow of CO_2 (should be 1–2L/min).
- Insert the laparoscope and evaluate for unexpected pathology and adhesions, particularly in the right upper quadrant between the gallbladder and omentum, transverse colon, and duodenum.
- Insert a second 10mm port 1cm below the xiphoid process via a transverse stab incision. Ensure that the port passes into the peritoneal cavity to the right of the falciform ligament.
- Insert two 5mm ports below the right costal margin – the first in the midclavicular line and the second in the anterior axillary line.

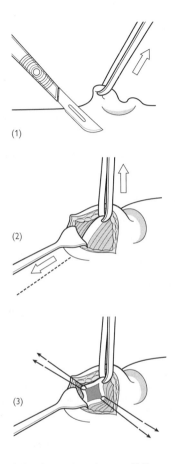

Fig. 10.6 Hasson technique for pneumoperitoneum. (1) Elevate umbilicus using Allis forceps. Make a 2cm transverse infra-umbilical incision. (2) Bluntly dissect onto linea alba staying in the midline. Elevate the linea alba using Kocker's forceps. Incise vertically through linea alba. (3) Insert stay sutures (3/0 vicryl) into linea alba. Penetrate parietal peritoneum by blunt dissection using closed tip of McIndoe's scissors. Insert blunt trocar and secure with stay sutures.

Dissecting Calot's triangle
- Beware of anatomical variations (see Box 10.1).
- With the patient in a reverse Trendelenburg position (30° head down) and rotated 15° to the left, grasp the gallbladder fundus with toothed grasping forceps, and lift the gallbladder cephalad.
- Separate adhesions using the diathermy hook, staying close to the gallbladder to avoid the duodenal cap.
- With a second grasper in the left hand, grasp Hartmanns pouch, and retract it to the right to open Calot's triangle (see Fig. 1.5).
- Using the diathermy hook, dissect the peritoneum overlying Calot's triangle.
- Staying close to the gallbladder wall, continue dissecting until the cystic duct and cystic artery can be identified with certainty. If the anatomy is unclear, convert to an open cholecystectomy.
- Apply three metal clips to both artery and duct (two clips on patient side) and divide these structures.
- If the cystic duct is too wide, apply an endoloop after performing a retrograde dissection of the gallbladder.

Intraoperative cholangiography
- Routinely performed in all patients by some surgeons.
- Selective use in cases of unclear anatomy or preoperative suspicion of CBD stones.
- Provides clear demonstration of the biliary anatomy and identifies stones in the common bile or hepatic ducts.
- After dissecting Calot's triangle, open the cystic duct with scissors and insert a cannula into the CBD.
- Inject contrast medium and view the cholangiogram on an image intensifier.
- On completion, ligate the cystic duct in the usual manner.

Removing the gallbladder
- Apply lateral traction on the gallbladder with the left hand.
- Dissect the gallbladder from the liver bed with the diathermy hook.
- Place the gallbladder into a laparoscopic retrieval bag, and remove via epigastric or umbilical port.
- Ensure haemostasis and wash out the peritoneal cavity with saline.
- Give IV cefuroxime 750mg if bile spillage during the procedure.
- Retrieve any spilt gallstones.
- Insert a 5mm suction drain into the subhepatic space in difficult cases.
- Remove ports under direct vision.
- Close the linea alba with 3/0 PDS.
- Close skin with 3/0 subcuticular monocryl.

Box 10.1 Anatomical variants encountered during laparoscopic cholecystectomy

Biliary
- Intrahepatic gallbladder.
- Duplication of gallbladder.
- Short cystic duct.
- Posterior sectoral duct.
- Accessory duct of Luschka.
- Narrow common bile duct.
- Low confluence of hepatic ducts.

Arterial
- Short cystic artery.
- Anterior and posterior cystic artery.
- Absent cystic artery.

Converting to open cholecystectomy

Indications
- Unsatisfactory progress.
- Unclear anatomy.
- CBD stones.
- Uncontrolled bleeding.
- Visceral or vascular injury.
- Bile duct injury.

Postoperative care
- Day case procedure or overnight stay.
- Regular analgesia and antiemetic.
- Oral fluids and diet as tolerated.
- Mobilize early.
- Remove drain (if inserted) after 12–24h unless ongoing bleeding or evidence of bile leak.
- If bile leak, record the daily volume. If persistent drainage and/or high volume, arrange an urgent MRCP and ERCP. Discuss with the regional hepatobiliary unit if common bile duct injury present.

Complications

Bleeding
- Presents with significant blood-stained output from drain, fall in haemoglobin, haemodynamic collapse, or secondary infection/sepsis.
- If patient hypotensive/shocked with evidence of significant bleeding (blood in drains, fall in haemoglobin), resuscitate/transfuse and arrange urgent laparotomy (Kocher's or midline incision).
- If patient stable, transfuse as necessary and arrange CT to exclude active arterial bleed, which may be amenable to angiographic embolization.
- Late haemorrhage (>7 days) likely to be due to a ruptured pseudoaneurysm.

Bile leak
- May be due to injury to accessory duct of Luschka, aberrant right posterior sectoral duct, divided, or injured CBD, or leak from cystic duct stump.
- May present with bile-stained fluid in drain (if inserted), abdominal pain, fevers, ileus, non-specific symptoms, or failure to progress.
- If large volume of bile-stained fluid in drain on first postoperative day, consider urgent laparoscopy to exclude cystic duct stump leak (may be treated by laparoscopic placement of clips).
- If patient is clinically unwell, shocked +/− peritonitic, consider urgent surgery (laparoscopy or laparotomy) to achieve adequate lavage and drainage.
- If low volume of bile drainage, arrange US/CT to exclude residual biloma, followed by ERCP if persistent.
- Diagnose bilomas by US/CT followed by percutaneous drainage.
- Give IV antibiotics and prophylactic antifungal therapy.
- For persistent bile leaks after 48–72h, ERCP and sphincterotomy (+/− CBD stent) will usually lead to resolution of small leaks. Cholangiographic evidence of injury to CBD, CHD, or RHD should prompt urgent referral to HPB unit. Arrange a CT angiogram to exclude a concomitant vascular injury.

Port-site hernia
- May presents in early postoperative period (<1 week) due to technical error. Abdominal pain (especially around port-site), vomiting, and distension, or non-specific symptoms and failure to progress.
- Late presentation with symptoms of hernia.
- Treat by open surgical repair +/− bowel resection if gangrenous.

Visceral/vascular injury
- Due to inadvertent injury during port placement, incorrect use of Verres needle, or off-screen injury (e.g. diathermy).
- May be evident at the time of laparoscopy or present in the early postoperative period. Treat by resuscitation and re-operation.

Carbon dioxide gas embolism
- Inadvertent insertion of Verres needle or port into periumbilical vein.
- Presents immediately with haemodynamic collapse.
- Prompt recognition essential to avoid adverse outcome.
- Position patient head down.
- Turn off CO_2 flow.

Wound infection
- Increased incidence if bile spillage intraoperatively or emergency cholecystectomy.
- Presents with wound pain, erythema, tenderness, or purulent discharge.
- Exclude incarcerated hernia (clinical assessment +/− US/CT).
- Treat by opening wound +/− antibiotics if cellulitis.

Open cholecystectomy

Indications
- Previous upper abdominal surgery.
- Pregnancy.
- Chronic obstructive airways disease (risk of pneumoperitoneum causing postoperative respiratory depression).
- Unsuccessful laparoscopic approach.
- Finding of gallbladder tumour at time of laparoscopy

Technique
- Kocher's incision (right subcostal).
- Grasp the gallbladder fundus with a Rampley's tissue holding forceps, lifting it cephalad.
- Perform a fundus-first dissection of the gallbladder.
- Dissect Calot's triangle using diathermy and right-angled forceps.
- Identify the cystic artery and duct, and ligate/divide them.
- If the structures in Calot's triangle cannot be safely identified (e.g. intense inflammation/fibrosis), perform a subtotal cholecystectomy by transecting the gallbladder through Hartmann's pouch. Close the gallbladder remnant using continuous 3/0 vicryl suture.

Post-operative care
- Open approach associated with longer hospital stay and delayed return to normal activities, compared to laparoscopic approach.
- Ensure adequate analgesia (e.g. epidural infusion or subcutaneous patient-controlled opiate analgesia).
- Postoperative care is otherwise similar to after laparoscopic cholecystectomy.
- Increased risk of cardiopulmonary complications, e.g. pneumonia.
- Uncomplicated hospital stay 3–4 days.

Complications
See Laparoscopic cholecystectomy 📖 p. 224.

Post-cholecystectomy problems

Causes
- Postoperative complication, e.g. bile leak, bile duct injury.
- Residual common bile duct stone.
- Alternative diagnosis, e.g. peptic ulcer.
- Post-cholecystectomy syndrome.

Assessment
- Take a careful history to determine whether the symptom (e.g. pain) was present before surgery or not.
- In some patients diagnosed with gallstones, the presenting symptom may not be typical for biliary colic, and may be due to another pathology. In such cases, the symptom will obviously persist after cholecystectomy. It is therefore vital to take a thorough history of the presenting complaint, particularly of the characteristics of the pain.
- If there is any suspicion that the patient's symptoms may not be due to gallstones, it is necessary to investigate for alternative causes (e.g. OGD, colonoscopy, CT scan) before considering cholecystectomy.
- Arrange US to exclude intra-abdominal abscess/bile leak and assess for biliary dilatation.
- Check LFTs.
- Consider MRCP if suspecting CBD stone.

Retained CBD stone after cholecystectomy
- Patients usually present with biliary colic +/– jaundice or abnormal LFTs.
- Stones should be removed by ERCP.

CBD stricture
- CBD strictures may develop after cholecystectomy due to:
  - scarring from previous cholangitis/CBD stones;
  - biliary stents;
  - ischaemic injury to CBD.
- Treat by endoscopic or percutaneous balloon dilatation and/or stenting. Perform Roux-en-Y hepaticojejunostomy for resistant, symptomatic strictures, not responsive to endoscopic measures.

Sphincter of Oddi dysfunction
- Biliary pain either due to dyskinesia or stenosis of sphincter of Oddi.
- Aetiology unknown.
- Endoscopic sphincter of Oddi manometry may confirm the diagnosis.
- **Sphincter of Oddi stenosis:** high basal pressures lead to biliary pain and/or pancreatitis.
- **Sphincter of Oddi dyskinesia**: manometry findings of excess retrograde contractions, spasm, paradoxical increase in sphincter contraction following CCK.
- **ERCP and sphincterotomy:** effectively relieves symptoms in the majority.

Post-cholecystectomy diarrhoea
- Incidence 10–20%.
- Aetiology is unknown, but may be due to malabsoprtion of bile acids and/or increased colonic transit times.
- Antidiarrhoeal agents (e.g. loperamide 4mg qds) are usually effective in controlling symptoms.

Iatrogenic bile duct injuries

Aetiology
- Estimated incidence 0.1%.
- Most occur as a result of *misidentification*, rather than inadequate knowledge or insufficient manual skill.

Prevention
The risk of bile duct injury (BDI) may be reduced by the following approaches:
- Use high quality imaging equipment.
- Find Calot's triangle early.
- Apply *lateral* traction on GB.
- Clear the medial wall of GB infundibulum.
- Clearly visualize cystic duct entering GB.
- Selective use of cholangiography, e.g. unclear anatomy, difficult dissection.
- Low threshold for converting to open procedure, e.g. reduced visibility due to bleeding.

Clinical presentation
- 75% of injuries are unrecognized at the time of surgery.
- **Intraoperative diagnosis:** bile leak.
- **Postoperative presentation:**
  - bile leak;
  - collection;
  - obstructive jaundice (due to ligation, division, or ischaemic damage);
  - secondary biliary cirrhosis.

For Bismuth and Strasberg classifications see Figs 10.7 and 10.8.

Management of bile duct injuries
Intraoperative diagnosis
- Contact hepatobiliary surgeon immediately.
- Depending on resources, the hepatobiliary unit may provide an outreach service, travelling to the referring hospital to perform primary repair, or arrange urgent transfer.

Postoperative bile leak and/or jaundice
- Drain sepsis (percutaneous or open).
- Arrange urgent cholangiogram (MRCP).
- Arrange urgent CT angiography to exclude co-existing vascular injury.
- Discuss with hepatobiliary unit.

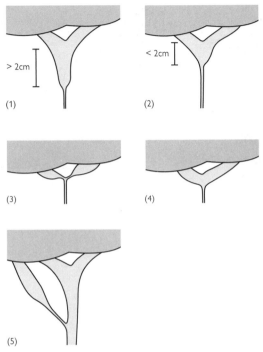

Fig. 10.7 Bismuth classification of biliary strictures. (1) >2cm from hepatic duct confluence. (2) <2cm from hepatic duct confluence. (3) At hepatic duct confluence. (4) Involving left or right hepatic duct. (5) Involving accessory hepatic duct.

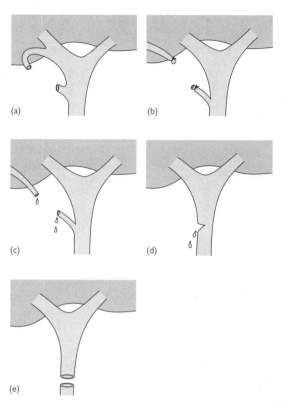

Fig. 10.8 Strasberg classification of iatrogenic bile duct injuries. (a) Leak from accessory hepatic duct. (b) Ligated accessory hepatic duct. (c) Leak from aberrant right posterior sectoral duct. (d) Lateral injury to common hepatic duct. (e) Injury to common hepatic/bile duct (subdivided according to Bismuth classification into E1–5).

Principles of treatment after transfer to hepatobiliary unit
- Treat sepsis.
- Stabilize patient (HDU or ITU).
- Review imaging (CT angiography, MRCP, or ERCP) to define anatomical location of injury.
- Plan definitive treatment.
- Long-term follow-up to exclude/treat biliary strictures.

Treatment options
- Depends on degree of duct and associated injuries.
- ERCP and stenting.
- Primary closure (+/– T-tube).
- Roux-en-Y hepaticojejunostomy.
- Hepatic resection.
- Orthotopic liver transplantation.

Complications after surgical treatment of bile duct injury
- Increased risk if surgery performed in the presence of sepsis, if associated vascular injury or if proximal injury.
- Biliary stricture.
- Abscess.
- Biliary fistula.
- Recurrent cholangitis.
- Secondary biliary cirrhosis.

Biliary atresia

- Incidence 1 per 12,000 live births.
- Associated congenital anomalies in up to 30% (e.g. situs inversus, gut malrotation, absence of retrohepatic vena cava, polysplenia/asplenia, preduodenal portal vein, Ladd's bands).
- Characterized by atrophy and fibrotic occlusion of both intra- and extrahepatic bile ducts.
- **Pathological findings:**
  - *early* – portal tract fibrosis, bile duct proliferation and bile stasis;
  - *late* – hepatocyte necrosis, inflammatory infiltrate;
  - histological features may be similar to alpha-1-antitrypsin deficiency.
- **Classification:**
  - *Type 1* – atresia of CBD +/– cystic dilatation (5%);
  - *Type 2* – atresia of common hepatic duct (3%);
  - *Type 3* – atresia of right and left hepatic ducts (>90%).
- Neonates present with obstructive jaundice, hepatosplenomegaly, vitamin K malabsorption, and failure to thrive.
- Assessment: history, examination, and basic investigations fail to distinguish between biliary atresia and other causes of neonatal jaundice (e.g. hepatitis, bile duct hypoplasia, choledochal cysts). Due to lack of intrahepatic bile duct dilatation in biliary atresia, US has limited value. Diagnosis of biliary atresia is made after excluding other disorders. Percutaneous liver biopsy is often useful (accuracy >80%).

Management

Type 1

- If gallbladder is patent and not shrunken, pre-operative diagnosis may be incorrect, and intraoperative cholangiography should be performed to confirm diagnosis of biliary atresia.
- Mobilize the liver.
- Perform cholecystectomy.
- Divide distal CBD.
- Perform retrocolic Roux-en-Y hepaticojejunostomy (single layer interrupted 5/0 PDS sutures).

Types 2 and 3

- Improved long-term results if Kasai portoenterostomy is performed within 8 weeks of birth.
- Mobilize the liver and gallbladder.
- Divide distal CBD.
- Dissect the hepatic duct from hepatic artery and portal vein.
- Excise bile duct tissue to the level of the liver capsule at the porta hepatis.
- Construct a 40cm retrocolic Roux-en-Y loop of jejunum.
- Anastomose Roux limb to liver hilum (interrupted 5/0 PDS).

Postoperative complications

- Incidence 40%.
- **Portal hypertension:** despite effective biliary drainage (either hepaticojejunostomy or portoenterostomy), hepatic fibrosis often progresses leading to portal hypertension. Bleeding from oesophageal varices is common and may be prevented by injection sclerotherapy, portsystemic shunt surgery, or transjugular intrahepatic portosystemic shunt. Liver transplantation may be indicated in refractory cases.
- **Recurrent jaundice:** exclude surgically treatable obstruction (radionuclide scan or percutaneous cholangiography). May be due to progressive liver disease. 50–60% of infants treated by portoenterostomy will have a good quality of life and normal serum bilirubin. The remainder should be considered for liver transplantation with good results (3-year survival 85%).

Gallbladder dyskinesia

- Biliary pain secondary to reduced or excessive contraction of the gallbladder. Aetiology unknown. Features similar to biliary colic with no US or MRCP evidence of gallstones.
- CCK cholescintigraphy may be helpful to confirm the diagnosis.
- Treatment is by cholecystectomy.

Pancreatic diseases

O. Tucker, R. Sutcliffe, & R. Deshpande

Acute pancreatitis

Incidence
- Increase in incidence in the past two decades.
- 3% of all admissions for abdominal pain.

Definition
- **Acute pancreatitis (AP):** an acute inflammatory process, with variable involvement of other regional tissues or remote organ systems.
- **Mild AP:** minimal organ dysfunction and uneventful recovery.
- **Severe AP:** organ failure +/− complications.

Aetiology
- **Toxic:** alcohol (*36% − percentages are incidences in developed countries), scorpion bite, organophosphate insecticide.
- **Gallstones:** increased incidence in white women aged ≥60 years. More frequent with small <5mm diameter gallstones (microlithiasis).
- **Idiopathic:** 15–25%.
- **Iatrogenic:** ERCP (diagnostic 1–3%, therapeutic 4–5%), major abdominal or cardiac surgery (coronary artery bypass).
- **Metabolic:** hyperlipidaemia (1–4%), hypercalcaemia.
- **Medication** (1·4–2%): asparaginase, pentamidine, azathioprine, steroids, cytarabine, didanosine, frusemide, sulfasalazine, mesalazine, sulindac, sulfamethoxazole-trimethoprim, mercaptopurine, tetracycline, opiates, valproic acid, pentavalent antimonials, oestrogens, paracetamol, hydrochlorothiazide, carbamazepine, interferon, cisplatin, lamivudine, cyclopenthiazide, octreotide, enalapril, phenformin, erythromycin, rifampicin.
- **Infectious:**
  - *viral* − mumps, CMV, EBV, coxsackie, Varicella zoster, hepatitis B, herpes, HIV;
  - *bacterial* − mycoplasma, legionella, leptospira, salmonella;
  - *parasitic* − ascaris, cryptosporidium, toxoplasma.
- **Obstructive:** biliary stone or sludge (38%), pancreatic or ampullary tumour, choledochal cyst, choledochocele, annular pancreas, pancreas divisum, focal pancreatic duct strictures due to prior blunt trauma or chronic pancreatitis (CP), sphincter of Oddi dysfunction, duodenal obstruction (duodenal diverticulum, Crohn's disease).
- **Autoimmune:** PAN, SLE, Sjogrens syndrome, PBC, PSC.
- **Genetic:** PRSS1, SPINK1, CFTR gene mutations.
- **Other causes:** trauma, hypothermia, repeated marathon running, pregnancy, ischaemia.

Pathogenesis

- Unregulated trypsin activation within pancreatic acinar cells leading to gland autodigestion and local inflammation.
- Intracellular protective mechanisms are overwhelmed, including trypsin synthesis as inactive enzyme trypsinogen, autolysis of activated trypsin, enzyme compartmentalization, specific trypsin inhibitor synthesis, serine protease inhibitor Kazal type 1 (SPINK1), and low intracellular ionized calcium.
- **Activation of elastase, phospholipase A2, complement + kinin pathways:** local production of inflammatory mediators; interleukin (IL) 1, IL6, IL8, TNFα. Endothelial cell activation, transendothelial leucocyte migration, further inflammatory mediator release.
- ↓ oxygen delivery and generation of oxygen-derived free radicals.
- Variable systemic inflammatory response syndrome progressing to multi-organ failure (MOF) +/− death.

Clinical presentation

Upper abdominal pain
- **Site:** central, epigastric.
- **Radiation:** directly through to the back.
- **Progression:** constant.
- **Duration:** 6–12h.
- **Severity:** severe pain 8–9/10.
- **Aggravating factors:** movement, lying supine.
- **Relieving factors:** leaning forward, analgesia.
- **Precipitating factors:** alcohol.

▶ In gallstone pancreatitis, the pain is typically sudden, epigastric, knife-like and may radiate to the back. In alcohol, metabolic, or hereditary causes the onset may be subacute with poorly localized pain.

Associated symptoms
- Anorexia.
- Nausea, vomiting.
- Pyrexia +/− rigors.

General examination

General inspection
- Level of distress.
- Cachexia.
- Jaundice.
- Alcohol factor.

Vital signs
Pyrexia, tachycardia, circulatory collapse, tachypnoea, renal failure.

Abdominal examination
- Tenderness in epigastrium/upper abdomen +/− peritonism +/− mass.
- **Cullen's sign:** periumbilical haemorrhagic discolouration.
- **Grey Turner sign:** haemorrhagic discolouration of the flanks

Investigations
- **Blood investigations:**
  - FBC;
  - U&E;
  - amylase (total and pancreatic specific), lipase;
  - LFT's;
  - glucose;
  - CRP;
  - calcium;
  - ABG/lactate;
  - trypsinogen-2;
  - trypsin 2-α 1 antrypsin complex.
- **Urine analysis:** amylase, trypsinogen activation peptide (TAP).
- **Serum amylase:**
  - ≥3× upper limit of normal with classic symptoms are usually diagnostic;
  - ≥3-fold ALT ↓ has a 95% PPV in diagnosing a gallstone aetiology;
  - 15–20% of patients have normal serum hepatic enzyme levels.
- **Chest X-ray:** left pleural effusion +/– atelectasis).
- **Abdominal X-ray:** sentinel loop, colon 'cut off' sign, gallstones.
- **Ultrasound** (gallstones/sludge, dilated CBD +/– intrahepatic biliary tree, intraductal calculi, pancreatic pseudocyst/mass lesion): since gallstones are a treatable cause of pancreatitis, if ultrasound is negative, it should be repeated (BSG guidelines). Two negative ultrasounds in a patients with no other risk factors for pancreatitis should be followed by an MRCP.
- CT of the abdomen should be arranged in patients with severe AP who fail to resolve between days 3 and 10, or where diagnosis is uncertain (see Table 11.1). Demonstrates presence of peripancreatic inflammation, presence/extent of pancreatic necrosis, peripancreatic collections.
- **MRI/MRCP or EUS:** investigation of suspected intraductal stones, pancreatic mass lesion, early pancreatic duct disruption.

Clinical course
- 80% of patients have mild disease with mortality <1%.
- Patients with severe AP have a mortality rate of 20–40%.
- Overall mortality of 10–15% unchanged in last 2 decades.

Predictors of severity
- **Atlanta criteria:** presence of any condition in main categories indicates severe AP (see Table 11.2).
- **Ransons score** ≥3 (see Table 11.3).
- **Imrie score** ≥3 (see Box 11.1).
- **Acute Physiology, Age and Chronic Health Evaluation (APACHE) II Score:** calculated from 12 routine physiological measurements during the first 24h after admission, age and previous health status. APACHE II score ≥8 on admission predicts mortality of 11–18%.
- CRP ≥150mg/dl at 24h.
- **Obesity:** BMI ≥30kg/m^2.

- **Haematocrit:** ≥44%.
- CT severity grade ≥6 (see Table 11.4).
- Persistent organ dysfunction within first 48h (see Tables 11.1–11.4, Box 11.1).
- Urinary TAP ≥35nmol/L.
- **Other serum measurements:** cytokines (interleukin 6 ≥400pg/mL on admission), phospholipase A2, PMN elastase >300μg/L, amyloid A, procalcitonin, TAP, trypsinogen 2.
- Polymorphism in chemokine monocyte chemotactic protein-1 (MCP-1).

Table 11.1 UK guidelines for the management of AP (2005). Available prognostic features that predict complications

In the first 24h	Clinical impression of severity
	Obesity
	APACHE II >8
After 48h	CRP >150mg/l
	Glasgow score >3
	Persisting organ failure

Table 11.2 Prediction of severe AP by the Atlanta criteria (Bradley 1993)

Criterion	Value
Ranson's score	>3
APACHE II score	>8
Organ failure	
Shock	Systolic blood pressure <90mmHg
Pulmonary insufficiency	Partial pressure of arterial oxygen <60mmHg
Renal failure	Creatinine >177μmol/L (2mg/dl) (after hydration)
Systemic complications	
Disseminated intravascular coagulation	Platelet count ≤100,000/mm3
	Fibrinogen level <1g/L
	Fibrin-split products >80μg/mL
Metabolic disturbance	Calcium ≤7.5mg/dL
Local complications	
Pancreatic necrosis	Present
Pancreatic abscess	Present
Pancreatic pseudocyst	Present

Table 11.3 Ranson's criteria

At presentation	Age	>55 years
	WBC	>16,000/mm^3
	Glucose	>10mmol/L (>200mg/dL)
	AST	>250iu/L
	LDH	>350iu/L
Within 48h	Arterial pO$_2$	<8kPa (<60mmHg)
	Blood urea nitrogen	>5mg/dL (1.8mmol/L) increase
	Calcium	<8mg/dL (2mmol/L)
	Base deficit	>4mEq/L
	Fluid sequestration	>6L
	Fall in haemocrit	>10%

Ransons score = 1 point for each factor. Predicted mortality based on score: 0–2 (3%), 3–4 (16%), 5–6 (40%), 7–8 (100%).

Box 11.1 Imrie (Glasgow) criteria

- WCC >15,000/mm^3.
- Glucose >10mmol/L.
- Urea >16.
- LDH >600iu/L.
- AST >200iu/L.
- Albumin <32g/dL.
- Calcium <2mmol/L.
- paO$_2$ <8kPa.

Imrie score = 1 point for each factor.

Management

Supportive
- Nil orally.
- Fluid resuscitation.
- Monitor fluid balance, respiratory and renal function, inflammatory parameters.
- Adequate analgesia.
- Stress ulcer prophylaxis.
- Manage in HDU or ITU for patients with impending or actual organ failure, significant comorbidity.

Table 11.4 CT severity index of acute pancreatitis (Balthazar 1990)

	Criterion	Value (points)
Unenhanced CT	Normal pancreas	0
	Pancreatic enlargement	1
	Intrinsic change; peripancreatic fat stranding	2
	Single, ill defined fluid collection	3
	Multiple fluid collections, or gas in or adjacent to pancreas	4
Contrast enhanced CT	0% necrosis	0
	30% necrosis	2
	30–50% necrosis	4
	>50% necrosis	6

Nutrition

- Early tube feeding enteral nutrition (EN) should be initiated in severe AP, particularly in malnourished alcoholics.
- Commence enteral feeding at 20ml/h with standard low fat (if tolerated) or peptide-based formulae. Increase to full volume within 48h
- EN down-regulates splanchnic cytokine production, modulates the acute phase response, reduces catabolism and preserves protein.
- Recent meta-analysis of 6 randomized trials: ↓ infection rates, ↓ surgical intervention, ↓ length of hospital stay, ↓ cost with EN.
- ESPEN guidelines on nutritional support in AP (2006):
  - in severe AP, supplementation by parenteral nutrition may be required, or when EN is contraindicated (e.g. prolonged ileus);
  - water, electrolyte, and micronutrient requirements must be met by the intravenous route and ↓ gradually as enteral supply increases;
  - the jejunal route is recommended if gastric feeding is not tolerated;
  - in severe AP with complications (fistula, ascites, pseudocyst) EN can be successfully performed;
  - in mild AP, EN has no positive impact on disease course. EN only recommended if cannot consume food after 5–7 days due to pain.

Prophylactic antibiotics

- The role of prophylactic antibiotic in severe AP is controversial.
- Current recommendations: give prophylactic antibiotics (e.g. 1g meropenem tds IV) for >30% necrosis and culture-proven infectious complications.
- If used, limit to 7–14 days (UK guidelines 2005).
- Several RCTs and meta-analyses have shown benefit in terms of reduced pancreatic or non-pancreatic infections, but results not widely reproduced. Mortality reduction not clear, but most studies inadequately powered.

Experimental therapies
- No proven benefit with inhibitors of the inflammatory response [platelet activating factor (PAF) inhibitor: lexipafant, PAF acetyl hydrolase, LI10, TNF antagonists), protease inhibitors (aprotinin,gabexate mesilate), or inhibition of pancreatic secretion with somatostatin or its analogues.
- Probiotic prophylaxis in predicted severe AP does not ↓ risk of infectious complications and is associated with ↑ risk of mortality (Dutch Acute Pancreatitis Study Group 2008).

ERCP
UK Guidelines on ERCP in Acute Gallstone Pancreatitis (2005): urgent therapeutic ERCP is recommended within the 72h after pain onset in severe AP of suspected or proven gallstone aetiology, or when there is cholangitis, jaundice (bilirubin > 90), or a dilated CBD. All require endoscopic sphincterotomy (ES) whether or not intraductal stones are found.

Timing of cholecystectomy
- For mild gallstone pancreatitis, perform cholecystectomy during index admission.
- For severe AP, wait until patient has clinically improved and inflammatory response/organ failure has resolved before performing cholecystectomy.

Complications of acute pancreatitis
- Peripancreatic fluid collection:
  - acute fluid collection;
  - pseudocyst;
  - organized pancreatic necrosis with surrounding fluid.
- Pancreatic abscess.
- Pancreatic necrosis.
- Infected pancreatic necrosis.
- Pseudoaneurysm.
- Segmental portal hypertension and variceal bleed (splenic +/– portal vein thrombosis).
- ARDS +/– MOF +/– death

See Fig. 11.1.

Acute fluid collections
- Occur early in the course of acute pancreatitis in or near the pancreas.
- Lack a wall of granulation tissue.
- May occur in up to 50% of cases of severe pancreatitis.
- 50% regress spontaneously within 6 weeks.
- 10–15% progress to pseudocyst formation after developing a capsule.
- Do not require treatment in an otherwise stable patient.
- Indications for intervention:
  - continuing enlargement with pain or adjacent organ compression;
  - infection. pain, pyrexia, leucocytosis, gas in fluid collection on CT;
  - treat by percutaneous drainage under US/CT guidance.

Acute pancreatic pseudocyst
- **Definition:** a collection of pancreatic juice within or adjacent to the pancreas enclosed by a wall of fibrous or granulation tissue.
- **Aetiology:** liquefaction of necrotic tissue, ductal disruption with leakage, ductal obstruction (stones, stricture in chronic pancreatits).
- Usually develop in the setting of chronic pancreatits (20–40%) due to ductal obstruction and disruption.
- Development of an acute pseudocyst takes ≥4 weeks from onset of AP.

PC are usually preceded by, and need to be distinguished from an acute peripancreatic fluid collection.

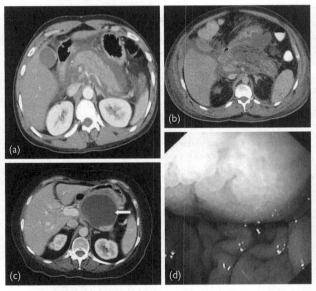

Fig. 11.1 Complications of acute pancreatitis. (a) Acute fluid collection. (b) Pancreatic necrosis. (c,d) CT and endoscopic appearances of a pseudocyst.

- There is overlap between a pseudocyst and organized pancreatic necrosis where solid material can be surrounded by fluid.
- A communication between the pseudocyst and pancreatic ductal system may be demonstrated radiologically in 80% at ERCP.
- Expectant management of acute asymptomatic pseudocysts regardless of size or duration. 50% will resolve within 6 weeks.
- **Clinical presentation:**
  - pain;
  - persistent fever with elevated serum amylase;
  - gastric outlet obstruction;
  - jaundice due to biliary obstruction;

- failure of resolution of AP;
- palpable epigastric mass.
- **Complications:**
  - infection;
  - haemorrhage;
  - obstruction of adjacent organs (stomach, bowel, ureters);
  - rapid expansion/rupture;
  - fistula.
- **Infection of pancreatic pseudocyst (<10%):**
  - usually with gut flora;
  - CT or USS guided catheter drainage successful in 85%;
  - percutaneous drainage less successful in loculated collections.
- **Rupture of a pancreatic pseudocyst (<3%):**
  - can be silent or present with severe pain;
  - can rupture into stomach, duodenum, colon, peritoneal, or pleural cavity causing pancreatic ascites or pleural effusion.
- Larger PCs are more likely to require operative drainage, but no absolute size criteria exist.

Management of persistent communicating PS
- Pancreatic sphincterotomy +/− stenting of the main pancreatic duct disruption. Leave stent in situ for 4–6 weeks.
- Recurrence rate 10–20%.

Management of non-communicating symptomatic PS
- Percutaneous radiologically guided drainage.
- **Indications:**
  - poor risk patient;
  - infected cyst in a septic patient;
  - immature cyst;
  - peripancreatic fluid collection;
  - unusually located cyst not amenable to internal drainage;
  - uncertain diagnosis where malignancy cannot be ruled out.
- **Outcome:**
  - recurrence (aspiration >70%, prolonged drainage 25%);
  - overall failure rate (aspiration 55%, drainage 30%).
- **Endoscopic or EUS-guided drainage:**
  - direct drainage (cystgastrostomy or cystduodenostomy);
  - indirect drainage (transpapillary);
  - complications. perforation, haemorrhage, infection, recurrence, stent blockage/migration.
- **Surgery (laparoscopic or open):**
  - direct drainage into upper gastrointestinal tract;
  - pancreatic resection if malignancy suspected.

Pseudoaneurysm
- Focal weakness of an artery due to infection and/or pancreatic leak.
- **Site:** splenic (45%), gastroduodenal (18%), or pancreaticoduodenal (18%) arteries.
- **Clinical presentation:** asymptomatic or rupture (intra-abdominal or gastrointestinal haemorrhage). May be preceded by low grade fever.

- Massive GI bleeding can result if the pseudoaneurysm communicates with the main pancreatic duct (haemosuccus pancreaticus).
- In patients with severe AP, CT scans should be performed at 7–10-day intervals to identify pseudoaneurysms prior to rupture.
- Treat by angio-embolization.
- Surgical intervention may be indicated in a critically unstable patient or where angiographic expertise unavailable.

Pancreatic abscess
- Circumscribed intra-abdominal collection of pus containing little or no necrosis, usually in proximity to the pancreas.
- Due to infection of an acute fluid collection or pseudocyst.
- Treat by percutaneous drainage.

Pancreatic necrosis
- Diffuse or focal areas of nonviable pancreatic parenchyma.
- Typically associated with peripancreatic fat necrosis.
- Diagnosed by loss of tissue perfusion on contrast-enhanced CT scan.
- Associated with significantly increased mortality.
- Infected pancreatic necrosis requires intervention. Sterile necrosis can usually be managed non-operatively, but clinical deterioration is an indication for intervention.

Infected pancreatic necrosis
- Increased mortality compared to sterile necrosis (25% vs. 10%).
- Suspect if unexplained clinical deterioration or progressive decline with pyrexia, leucocytosis, and rising inflammatory markers.
- Diagnosed by presence of gas within necrotic tissue on contrast enhanced CT.
- In cases of uncertainty, consider fine needle aspiration, and culture of the necrotic area.
- Treat with appropriate antibiotics and drainage +/– debridement
- Early surgery (within 2 weeks) carries high mortality due to risk of bleeding and fistula. Improved outcome if surgical debridement delayed until >2 weeks.

Treatment options for infected pancreatic necrosis
- Open necrosectomy and drainage +/– packing +/– closed lavage.
- Lateral retroperitoneal approach.
- Minimally invasive retroperitoneal approach.
- Laparoscopic necrosectomy.
- USS- or CT-guided wide bore percutaneous catheter drainage with delayed necrosectomy.

Further information

Balthazar, E.J., Robinson, D.L., Megibow, A.J., & Ranson, J.H. (190) Acute pancreatitis: value of CT in establishing prognosis. *Radiology* **174**, 331–6.

Besselink, M.G., van Santvoort, H.C., Buskens, E., Boermeester, M.A., van Goor, H., Timmerman, H.M., Nieuwenhuijs, V.B., Bollen, T.L., van Ramshorst, B., Witteman, B.J., Rosman, C., Ploeg, R.J., Brink, M.A., Schaapherder, A.F., Dejong, C.H., Wahab, P.J., van Laarhoven, C.J., van der Harst, E., van Eijck, C.H., Cuesta, M.A., Akkermans, L.M., Gooszen, H.G., and the Dutch Acute Pancreatitis Study Group. (2008) Probiotic prophylaxis in predicted severe acute pancreatitis: a randomised, double-blind, placebo-controlled trial. *Lancet* **371**(9613), 651–9.

Bradley, E.L. 3rd. (1993) A clinically based classification system for acute pancreatitis. Summary of the International Symposium on Acute Pancreatitis, Atlanta, Ga, September 11–13, 1992. *Arch Surg* **128**, 586–90.

Chronic pancreatitis

Definition
- Progressive chronic irreversible inflammatory process of the pancreas.
- Histological evidence of inflammation and fibrosis.
- Eventual destruction of exocrine and endocrine tissue.

Incidence
3–9 cases/100,000 population.

Sex
- M: F 7:3 (per 100,000 population).
- Alcohol-induced chronic pancreatitis (CP) is more prevalent in males.
- Idiopathic and hyperlipidemic-induced CP is more prevalent in females.
- Equal sex ratios are observed in CP associated with hereditary pancreatitis.

Age
- Mean age at diagnosis. 46 ± 13 years.
- Bi-modal age distribution in idiopathic CP.
- **Early onset:** median age 19.2 years.
- **Late onset:** median age 56.2 years.

Survival rates
- 10-year survival rate = 70%.
- 20-year survival rate = 45%.

Classification
- **1963 Marseille classification:**
  - *acute pancreatitis* – acute, acute recurrent;
  - *chronic pancreatitis* – chronic, chronic relapsing.
- **1983 Cambridge classification:** chronic pancreatitis – chronic calcific-alcohol related, chronic obstructive (Table 11.5).
- ICD classification.

Aetiology
Alcohol (60%)
- Abnormalities of the pancreatic protease/protease inhibitor system may play a role in its pathogenesis.
- The serine protease inhibitor Kazal type I (SPINK1) gene (N34S) mutation was reported in 5.8% of patients with alcoholic CP vs. 1% of non-alcohol-related CP.

Idiopathic (10–30%)
A combination of calcium-sensing receptor (CASR) and SPINK1 gene mutations have been proposed to predispose to idiopathic CP.

Congenital
- Pancreas divisum with minor papilla stenosis.
- Annular pancreas divisum. Disease process involves the dorsal pancreas only.

Table 11.5 Cambridge grading of chronic pancreatitis by ERCP

Grade	Main pancreatic duct	Side branches
Normal	Normal	Normal
Equivocal	Normal	<3 abnormal
Mild	Normal	=3 abnormal
Moderate	Abnormal	>3 abnormal
Severe	Abnormal + ≥ 1 of: Large cavity (10mm) Duct obstruction Intraductal filling defect Severe duct dilatation or irregularity	>3 abnormal

Obstructive (10%)
Acquired
- Traumatic pancreatic duct stricture.
- Pancreatic duct stricture after acute necrotizing pancreatitis.
- Benign pancreatic duct obstruction.
- Sphincter of Oddi stenosis or dysfunction.
- Pancreatic, ampullary, or duodenal carcinoma.

Autoimmune
- Isolated autoimmune CP.
- Associated with autoimmune diseases, e.g. Sjögren's syndrome, primary biliary cirrhosis.
- Autoimmune chronic pancreatitis can mimic pancreatic carcinoma clinically and radiologically, and may be diagnosed on postoperative histology.
- **Histological subtypes:** lymphoplasmacytic sclerosing pancreatitis or idiopathic duct-destructive pancreatitis.
- Diagnosis suspected if elevated serum IgG4.
- **Confirm diagnosis by needle biopsy:** moderate to marked infiltration by IgG4-positive plasma cells (>10/HPF), particularly in the lymphoplasmacytic sclerosing pancreatitis subtype.
- Treat with high dose corticosteroids.

Tropical
- Tropical calcific pancreatitis.
- Fibrocalculous pancreatic diabetes. Seen in tropical countries in young non-alcoholic patients who are often malnourished.
- CASR mutations may be implicated in tropical chronic pancreatitis (TCP), and the risk may be increased with an associated SPINK1 mutation. CASR mutations have been demonstrated in 22% of patients with TCP, with a combination of both SPINK1 (N34S) and CASR mutations in 6%.

Genetic
- **Hereditary pancreatitis (1%):** autosomal dominant disorder with 80% penetrance. Mutations in the cationic trypsinogen (PRSS1) (R122H in 3rd exon) and SPINK1 (mutation N34S) genes have been linked to hereditary CP. PRSS1 mutations increase autocatalytic conversion of trypsinogen to active trypsin. SPINK1 is a potent protease inhibitor preventing premature intrapancreatic activation of trypsin and pancreatic autodigestion
- **Cystic fibrosis <1%:** autosomal recessive disorder. Associated with cystic fibrosis transmembrane conductance regulator (CFTR)-gene mutations. Range of clinical manifestations depending on the extent of the gene mutation.

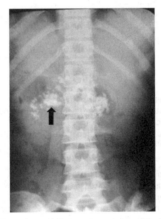

Fig. 11.2 Chronic pancreatitis. Plain X-ray appearances of chronic pancreatitis showing pancreatic calcification (arrowed).

Metabolic
- Hypercalcaemia (due to primary hyperparathyroidism). A combination of hypercalcemia and genetic variants in SPINK1 or CFTR increase the risk of primary hyperparathyroidism-related CP.
- Hyperlipidaemia. Inherited (Types I and V) or acquired.

Other causes
- Drugs.
- Radiotherapy.

Pathophysiology
- Toxic-metabolic hypothesis.
- Ductal obstruction hypothesis.
- Oxidative stress hypothesis.
- Necrosis-fibrosis hypothesis.

- Ischaemia hypothesis.
- Autoimmune.
- Genetic hypothesis:
  - CFTR mutation(s);
  - cationic trypsinogen gene mutation(s);
  - SPINK1 gene mutations.

Histopathological features
- Lymphocyte, plasma cell, and macrophage infiltration.
- Interlobular fibrosis.
- Intraductal eosinophilic plugs.
- Replacement of acinar cells by fibrosis.
- Progressive pancreatic ductal destruction.
- Calcification of protein plugs.
- Islet cells are preserved until very late in the process.

Clinical presentation
- Abdominal +/− back pain:
  - *majority* – intermittent attacks of severe pain lasting several hours;
  - *minority* – chronic often severe pain;
  - *location* – mid- or left upper abdomen, interscapular, occasionally band-like.
- Often long delay between symptom onset and diagnosis.
- Mean time to diagnosis = 62 ± 4 months.
- Mean time to diagnosis in alcohol-related CP = 81 months.
- Impairment of exocrine function: steatorrhea.
- Signs of exocrine insufficiency not apparent until 90% of gland destroyed.
- Impairment of endocrine function (diabetes mellitus).
- Weight loss. Fear of eating due to postprandial pain or exocrine insufficiency with malnutrition.
- **Complications of CP:**
  - *jaundice* – stricture of intrapancreatic portion of common bile duct.
  - *gastrointestinal bleeding* – gastric varices and left-sided portal hypertension due to splenic vein thrombosis;
  - *gastrointestinal obstruction* – duodenal stricture;
  - *pseudocyst formation* – symptoms determined by site and nature
  - *pain* – expansion, compression of adjacent structures, infection with abscess formation, rupture into adjacent cavities, or viscera with fistula formation;
  - *pancreatic ascites* – disrupted pancreatic duct.
  - pleural effusion;
  - pericardial effusion;
  - *gastrointestinal bleed* – rupture of pseudoaneurysm of the splenic, common hepatic, gastroduodenal, or pancreaticoduodenal arteries.

Patient evaluation
- Take a careful history with special reference to risk factors, complications and presence of pancreatic exocrine or endocrine dysfunction (see Chronic pancreatitis, Aetiology, clinical presentation).
- Diagnosis made by combination of clinical and radiological features.

- **Anatomical studies:**
  - abdominal X-ray;
  - CT abdomen;
  - MRI pancreas;
  - EUS (Table 11.6);
  - ERCP.
- Radiological findings (Table 11.7):
  - parenchymal calcification;
  - duct derangement (e.g. chain of lakes);
  - parenchymal cysts;
  - focal mass.
- **Functional assessment:**
  - *serum amylase, lipase* – typically normal or mildly elevated
  - *serum trypsin* – low in advanced CP;
  - *serum glucose*;
  - faecal human pancreatic elastase 1 and chymotripsin analysis;
  - direct function tests after hormonal stimulation: secretin, secretin-cholecystokinin, Lundh test;
  - *indirect function tests* – N-benzoyl-l-tyrosyl-*p*-aminobenzoic acid (NBT-PABA) test, pancreolauryl test, faecal fat estimation.

Table 11.6 Diagnosis of chronic pancreatitis by endoscopic ultrasonography

Ductal features	Main pancreatic duct dilation
	Duct irregularity
	Hyperechoic pancreatic ductal margins
	Dilated side branches
	Pancreatic duct stones
Parenchymal features	Hyperechoic foci
	Hyperechoic strands
	Lobularity of contour of gland
	Cysts

Table 11.7 Grading of chronic pancreatitis by abdominal US or CT

Normal	No abnormality seen on a good quality study with visualization of the entire gland
Equivocal	Mild pancreatic duct dilation (2–4 mm) in the body of the gland or Pancreatic gland enlargement ≤ twice normal
Mild to moderate	Equivocal grade plus ≥ one of the following: Pancreatic duct dilation Pancreatic duct irregularity Cavities <10mm diameter Parenchymal heterogeneity Increased echogenicity of wall of pancreatic duct Irregular contour of pancreatic head or body Focal parenchymal necrosis
Severe	Mild/moderate grade plus ≥ one of the following: Cavity >10mm diameter Intraductal filling defects Calculi/pancreatic calcification Ductal obstruction (stricture) Severe duct dilation or irregularity Contiguous organ involvement

Management
- 30–50% do not respond to conservative management and become opioid dependent.
- Abstinence from alcohol and smoking.

Dietary measures
- **Daily allowance:** 2000–3000 calories, low fat (20–25% of total calories), high protein (1.5–2g/kg), high carbohydrate (5–6g/kg).
- **ESPEN guidelines:** over 80% can be adequately treated with normal food supplemented with pancreatic enzymes. 10–15% require nutritional supplements and 5% require tube feeding.
- Exogenous fat-soluble vitamins (A,D,E,K).
- Exogenous vitamin B12.

Medical
- Gastric acid suppression.
- Treat exocrine insufficiency – enzyme replacement (e.g. Creon) with food. Medium chain triglyceride diet in patients with severe fat malabsorption.
- Treat diabetes.

Pain control
- Simple analgesics (e.g. paracetamol, NSAIDs).
- Opioids (e.g. tramadol, morphine).
- Bilateral thorascopic splanchnicectomy.
- EUS-guided coeliac plexus blockade.

Endoscopic therapy
- The aim is to decompress an obstructed pancreatic duct to relieve pain.
- **Indications:**
  - papillary stenosis;
  - pancreatic duct stricture;
  - pancreatic duct stones;
  - pancreatic pseudocyst.
- **Procedures:**
  - pancreatic duct sphincterotomy;
  - transpapillary stent;
  - pancreatic duct stricture dilation and stent placement;
  - pancreatic duct stone extraction +/– preprocedural extracorporealshockwave lithotripsy (ESWL);
  - transgastric/transduodenal pseudocyst drainage +/– stent.

Surgical management of chronic pancreatitis
Indications for surgery
- Intractable pain.
- Complications of chronic pancreatitis.
- Suspected pancreatic carcinoma.

Surgical options
- **Resection:**
  - Whipple's (classic or pylorus preserving pancreatico-duodenectomy);
  - spleen-preserving distal pancreatectomy (unless splenic vein thrombosis);
  - subtotal pancreatectomy;
  - total pancreatectomy.
- **Drainage procedure:** Partington-Rochelle longitudinal pancreatico-jejunostomy.
- **Combined resection and drainage:**
  - duval pancreatico-jejunostomy;
  - Puestow-Gillesby pancreatico-jejunostomy;
  - Frey's procedure;
  - Beger's procedure.
- **Neuroablative techniques.**
- **Transplant options:**
  - Islet autotransplantation;
  - segmental pancreatic autotransplantation;
  - pancreas allotransplantation.

Selection of surgical procedure
- Depends on:
  - general fitness of patient;
  - presence of comorbidity;
  - duration of symptoms;
  - predominant symptoms (e.g. pain, jaundice, diabetes);
  - anatomical factors (e.g. dilated pancreatic duct, focal mass);
  - experience of surgeon.

Results of surgery
- In well-selected patients, surgery (resection and/or drainage) can achieve effective pain relief (freedom from opiates) in 80–85% in experienced centres and significantly reduce incidence of acute exacerbations.
- Short-term results appear to be superior following the Beger procedure compared to Whipple's, but there is no difference in long-term results.

Pancreatic tumours

Definition of location
- **Head:** arising to the right of the left border of the superior mesenteric vein (SMV). The uncinate process is part of the head.
- **Body:** arising between the left border of the SMV and the left border of the aorta.
- **Tail:** arising between the left border of the aorta and the hilum of the spleen.

Classification
Primary
Epithelial
- Exocrine (>90% of all malignant pancreatic tumours).
- Endocrine.
- Combined.
- Epithelial tumours with uncertain differentiation:
  - solid pseudopapillary;
  - pancreaticoblastoma;
  - undifferentiated carcinoma.

Non-epithelial
- Angioma.
- Lymphoma.
- Lipoma, liposarcoma.
- Histiocytoma, malignant histiocytoma.
- Malignant lymphoma.
- Leiomyoma, leiomyosarcoma.
- Paraganglioma.
- Fibroma, fibrosarcoma.
- Rhabdomyosarcoma.
- Osteogenic sarcoma.
- Malignant schwannoma.

Metastatic
- Breast.
- Malignant melanoma.
- Lung.
- Renal cell carcinoma.

Primary malignant tumours of the exocrine pancreas

Histopathologic types

- Severe ductal dysplasia/carcinoma *in situ*.
- Ductal adenocarcinoma (>90%).
- Mucinous non-cystic carcinoma.
- Signet ring carcinoma.
- Adenosquamous carcinoma.
- Undifferentiated (anaplastic) carcinoma.
- Mixed (ductal-endocrine or acinar-endocrine) carcinoma.
- Osteoclast-like giant cell tumour.
- Cystadenocarcinoma (serous and mucinous types).
- Intraductal papillary mucinous carcinoma (IPMT).
- Invasive papillary mucinous carcinoma.
- Acinar cell carcinoma.
- Acinar cell cystadenocarcinoma.
- Small cell carcinoma.
- Pancreaticoblastoma.
- Solid pseudopapillary carcinoma.
- Papillary-cystic neoplasm (Frantz tumour).
- Unclassified.

Pancreatic adenocarcinoma

Epidemiology
- UK incidence 6000 cases per year.
- 8–12/100,000 population per year.
- Worldwide ~200,000 cases per year.
- 13th commonest cancer incidence.
- 50% present with metastatic disease.
- 35% present with locally advanced disease.
- Resection is the only chance for cure.
- Only 10–20% with head and less than 3% of body/tail cancers are candidates for resection.
- Overall, median survival is 4.4 months, and 5-year survival is 9.7%.
- After potentially curative resection, median survival is 12 months, and 5-year survival rate is 15–26%.

Risk factors
- **Age:** 80% of patients diagnosed age 70–80 years. 1% diagnosed age <40 years.
- **Sex:** more common in women than men.
- **Race:** more common in African Americans, less common in Asian Americans than whites.
- **Smoking:** 10× the relative risk if >2 packs/day.
- Alcohol, coffee, high fat high protein low fibre diet.
- **Chronic pancreatitis:** 5–15 fold ↑ risk.
- Hereditary pancreatitis associated with 50–70-fold ↑ risk.
- **Diabetes mellitus:** 2× relative risk diabetic onset >3 years before diagnosis. 3× relative risk diabetic onset >2 years before diagnosis.
- **Abdominal surgery:** 2–5× the relative risk. Prior partial gastrectomy, cholecystectomy.
- **Occupational:** napthylamine, ethyl dichloride, benzidine, metal-gas workers, chemists.
- **Hereditary** (see Pancreatic adenocarcinoma, Genetics).

Genetics
- 7–10% of pancreatic carcinoma related to genetic factors (see Tables 11.8–11.10).
- Several well-defined genetic syndromes of familial pancreatic cancer (FPC).
- No specific genetic mutations identified for the majority of FPC (70%).
- Relatives of FPC kindreds have a high risk of pancreatic cancer.

Pathophysiology
- Associated with an accumulation of mutations with progressive morphological changes.
- Current model proposes a progression from normal cuboidal to low columnar epithelium through a series of lesions termed pancreatic intraepithelial neoplasia (PanIN) to invasive carcinoma.

Table 11.8 Syndromic familial pancreatic cancer

Genetic syndrome	Germline mutation
Hereditary pancreatitis	PRSS1
HNPCC (Lynch II)	hMSH2, hMLH1
Familial breast cancer	BRAC-2
FAMMM syndrome	P16
FAP	APC
Peutz-Jeghers syndrome	STK11/LKB

Table 11.9 Non-syndromic familial pancreatic cancer (Tersemette 2001)

Pancreatic cancer	Family status	Estimated risk	Data set
Familial	2 relatives affected	18× ↑ risk	150 families
	3 relatives affected	57× ↑ risk	52 families
Sporadic		No ↑ risk	191 families

Table 11.10 Frequency of mutations in pancreatic cancer

Mutation	Incidence (%)
K-ras2	95
P16/CDKN2A	80
P21	75–85
TP53	50–75
Cyclin D1	95
DPC4/MADH4	55
Telomerase	95
BRCA-2	7–10
LKB1/STK11, MKK4, TGFβ I/II, RB1	5

Clinical features
- Non-specific symptoms (e.g. anorexia, nausea, bloating, weight loss, depression, change in bowel habit, dyspepsia, early satiety, fever, gastrointestinal bleed, intolerance to food, wine, tobacco, malaise, new-onset diabetes, pruritus, pyrosis, skin rashes/changes, sleep disorder).
- Classical presentation is with painless, progressive obstructive jaundice.
- Dull, vague, constant upper abdominal pain.
- Back pain (particularly with locally advanced disease).
- Acute pancreatitis.
- Gastric outlet obstruction.
- Cachexia or evidence of recent weight loss.
- Jaundice.

- Migratory thrombophlebitis (Trousseau's sign).
- Palpable abdominal mass.
- Hepatomegaly.

Investigations
- Blood tests. FBC, U/E, LFTs, amylase, Ca19.9.
- Transabdominal USS.
- Pancreatic protocol helical CT abdomen. Predicts resectability 80–90%, demonstrates local extension (see Box 11.2).
- MRCP.
- MRA/V: if suspected vascular invasion on CT.
- PET to exclude metastatic disease.
- EUS to assess vascular involvement and nodal status +/– fine needle aspiration cytology.
- Staging laparoscopy, intraoperative US and peritoneal cytology (see Box 11.3). Peritoneal cytology is not practiced widely, but may improve accuracy of staging and avoid unnecessary surgery in patients with occult peritoneal disease in up to 10%.

Preoperative staging
- AJCC TNM staging system (see Boxes 11.4 & 11.5).
- JPS (Japanese Pancreatic Society) classification. Similar to TNM except lymph node groups clearly defined (see Box 11.6).

Box 11.2 CT criteria of resectability of pancreatic cancer
- No extrapancreatic disease.
- No direct tumour extension to the coeliac axis or superior mesenteric artery (SMA).
- A patent SMV-PV confluence.

Box 11.3 Criteria for unresectability at staging laparoscopy
- Histologically confirmed hepatic, serosal, peritoneal, or omental metastases.
- Extrapancreatic extension of tumour, e.g. mesocolic involvement.
- Histologically confirmed coeliac or high portal node tumour involvement.
- Invasion or encasement of the coeliac axis, hepatic artery, or SMA.

Box 11.4 AJCC TNM staging of pancreatic cancer

T0: no evidence of primary tumour.
Tis: carcinoma *in situ*.
T1: tumour limited to the pancreas, $\leq$2cm in greatest diameter.
T2: tumour limited to the pancreas, >2 cm in greatest diameter.
T3: tumour extends beyond pancreas but no involvement of coeliac axis or superior mestenteric artery (SMA).
T4: tumour involves the coeliac axis or SMA (unresectable).
N0: no regional lymph node metastasis.
N1: regional lymph node metastasis.
M0: no distant metastasis.
M1: distant metastasis.

Stage 0	Tis	N0	M0	Localized within pancreas
Stage IA	T1	N0	M0	Localized within pancreas
Stage 1B	T2	N0	M0	Localized within pancreas
Stage IIA	T3	N0	M0	Locally invasive, resectable
Stage IIB	T1–3	N1	M0	Locally invasive, resectable
Stage III	T4 any	N	M0	Locally advanced, unresectable
Stage IV	Any T	Any N	M1	Distant metastases

Box 11.5 Regional lymph nodes in AJCC system*

- Peripancreatic, hepatic artery, superior mesenteric, retroperitoneal, lateral aortic.
- Infra-pyloric, coeliac (for tumours in head).
- Pancreaticolienal, splenic (for tumours in body/tail).

*Involvement of other nodal groups is considered metastastic.

Box 11.6 Lymph node groups according to JPS system

Group	Head carcinoma	Body-tail carcinoma
1	13a, 13b, 17a, 17b	8a, 8p, 10, 11p, 11d, 18
2	6, 8a, 8p, 12a, 12b,12p, 14p,14d	7, 9, 14p, 14d, 15
3	1, 2, 3, 4, 5, 7, 9, 10, 11p, 11d, 15, 16a2, 16b1, 18	5, 6, 12a, 12b, 12p, 13a, 13b, 17a, 17b, 16a2, 16b1

1. Right cardial; 2. left cardial; 3. lesser curvature stomach; 4. greater curvature stomach;
5. suprepyloric; 6. infrapyloric; 7. left gastric artery; 8. common hepatic artery; 9. coeliac artery;
10. splenic hilum; 11. splenic artery; 12. hepatoduodenal ligament; 13. posterior surface of head;
14. superior mesenteric artery; 15. middle colic artery; 16. abdominal aorta; 17. anterior surface
of head; 18. inferior margin of body-tail.

Management options
Resectable disease (Stages I–II)
Surgical resection +/– adjuvant chemotherapy or chemoradiotherapy.

Locally advanced unresectable disease (Stage III)
- Neoadjuvant chemoradiotherapy then re-staging CT +/– resection if down-staged.
- Palliative chemotherapy: 5-FU, folinic acid, and gemcitabine.
- Palliative chemoradiotherapy.
- Palliation of biliary and gastric outlet obstruction. Endoscopic or percutaneous metal stent. Surgical bypass (hepaticojejunostomy or gastrojejunostomy) if endoscopic/percutaneous methods fail and patient fit for surgery. Open or laparoscopic techniques depending on expertise.

Metastatic disease (Stage IV)
- Palliative chemotherapy (gemcitabine).
- Best supportive care.
- Pain control. Consider coeliac plexus block.
- Palliation of biliary and gastric outlet obstruction (as above).

Surgical resection
Resectability
- A tumour is potentially resectable if it can be technically removed with negative margins (R0 resection) without compromising the vascular supply to the liver (hepatic artery) or small bowel (superior mesenteric artery).
- Involvement of adjacent organs (e.g. duodenum or transverse colon), regional lymph nodes, portal vein (partial involvement), gastroduodenal artery are *not* contraindications to resection, as these structures can be removed *en bloc* with the tumour to achieve an R0 resection.
- A tumour is unresectable in the presence of:
  - major comorbidity;
  - metastatic disease (including involved lymph nodes outwith the resection field);
  - locally advanced disease with extrapancreatic involvement;
  - superior mesenteric artery or coeliac artery involvement;
  - main portal venous occlusion/thrombosis – PV encasement with occlusion and thrombosis is a contraindication to resection because arterial involvement is likely to co-exist.

Selection of procedure
Tumour in head of pancreas
- Whipple's pancreaticoduodenectomy (PD).
- Pylorus preserving pancreaticoduodenectomy (PPPD).
- PD with *en bloc* vascular resection and reconstruction.
- Tumour in body/tail:
  - distal pancreatectomy;
  - total pancreatctomy.

Favourable prognostic features
- Negative resection margin.
- Negative lymph nodes.
- Well/moderately differentiated carcinoma.
- Primary <2cm diameter.
- No perineural or lymphovascular invasion.

Portal vein resection
- Historically, portal vein involvement was a contraindication to resection. However, PV or SMV involvement is now considered to be related to tumour location, rather than biological behaviour.
- In 1973, Fortner described 'regional pancreatectomy'.
- *En bloc* resection of peripancreatic soft tissue, regional lymph nodes with portal vein resection (Type I) or resection/reconstruction of a major artery (Type II).
- Early results were poor (morbidity 67%, mortality 23%) with 3% 3-year survival.
- Portal vein resection is associated with longer operating time, increased blood loss, increased perioperative morbidity, and mortality compared to standard PD.
- Regional pancreatectomy is now associated with <4% mortality, 26% 5–year survival and reduced morbidity in high volume centres, due to:
  - advances in radiological and surgical techniques;
  - improved staging;
  - better patient selection;
  - adjuvant chemotherapy.
- Resection margins (R0 vs. R1/R2) and lymph node status are more important than portal vein involvement *per se* in terms of long-term survival. PD with PV resection has similar survival compared to standard PD (in absence of SMA or coeliac axis involvement).
- PD with PV resection should only be performed at centres with expertise in complex pancreatic surgery and only if an R0 resection can be achieved.
- Resected PV can be replaced if necessary with internal jugular or saphenous interpositional vein graft (see Fig. 11.3).

Superior mesenteric artery or coeliac axis involvement
- Contraindication to resection.
- Predicts extensive mesenteric neural plexus involvement and an inability to achieve a negative retroperitoneal margin even with radical surgery.
- Arterial resection and reconstruction is associated with a high operative mortality and morbidity with poor long-term outcome.
- Standard or extended resection with a grossly positive retroperitoneal margin has a median survival of <1 year.
- 60% with invasion of the tunica intima have extrapancreatic nerve plexus involvement.

Extended vs. standard lymphadenectomy

- Several centres have reported a survival benefit with extended lymphadenectomy ('standard' *plus* resection of lymph nodes along arterial supply) compared with standard lymphadenectomy (resection of peripancreatic, periduodenal, and perigastric lymph nodes).
- Data from RCTs and a meta-analysis do not show any benefit, and there is potentially increased morbidity with extended lymphadenectomy.
- Extended lymphadenectomy cannot be recommended outside of adequately powered RCTs.

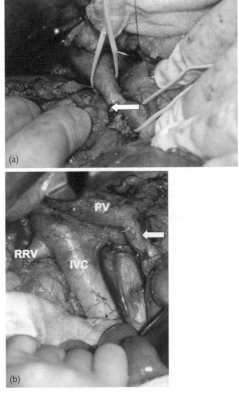

Fig. 11.3 Portal vein resection. (a) Operative images of an uncinate process tumour invading the portal vein, which required segmental resection (b, arrowed) to achieve a negative resection margin. PV: portal vein, IVC: inferior vena cava, RRV: right renal vein.

Cystic lesions

Classification

Inflammatory
- Pseudocyst (80%).
- Retention cyst (cystic fibrosis).

Congenital
- Solitary/multiple cysts (von Hippel Lindau).
- Lymphoepithelial cyst.
- Polycystic kidney disease.
- Medullary cystic kidney.
- Duplication cysts.
- Duodenal diverticulae.
- Familial fibrocystic pancreatic atrophy.
- CMV infection.

Tumours
- Mucinous cystadenoma.
- Serous cystadenoma.
- Mucinous cystadenocarcinoma.
- Endothelial tumour.
- Intraductal papillary mucinous tumour (IPMT).
- Intraductal oncocytic papillary tumour (subtype of IPMT).
- Solid pseudo-papillary tumour (SPPT).
- Cystic change in typically solid tumours.
- Pleomorphic carcinoma.
- Islet cell tumour.
- Acinar cell cystadenoma.
- Cystadenocarcinoma.
- Cystic teratoma.
- Cystic metastases.
- Cystic schwannoma.

Vascular
- Haemangioma.
- Angiosarcoma.
- Lymphangioma.
- Pancreatoblastoma.
- Epidermoid cysts within intrapancreatic accessory spleen.
- Dermoid cyst.

Peripancreatic
- Mesenteric cyst.
- Paraduodenal wall cyst.

Miscellaneous
- Parasitic.
- Necrotic tuberculous infection.
- Cystic change in amyloidosis.
- Endometriotic cysts.

Investigations

- Benign cystadenomas (serous or mucinous) and cystadenocarcinoma are the most common cystic tumour and account for 75% of cases.
- The aims of investigation are to confirm pancreatic origin, exclude pseudocyst, and determine the probability of malignancy (which require resection).
- **Blood tests:** FBC, LFTs, amylase, serum CA19.9, serum CEA.
- US/CT.
- MRCP.
- ERCP and cytology.
- **EUS and FNA:** send cyst fluid for biochemical analysis (CEA, CA19.9, CA72.4, CA15.3, amylase) and cytology.

Serous cystadenoma

- 32% of cystic tumours.
- Microcystic appearance >6 cysts of <2cm maximal diameter central calcification +/− enhancement around microcysts or of septa +/− larger cysts around periphery.
- EUS demonstrates microcystic component in tumours ≤3cm diameter.
- Macrocystic forms in 10%.
- **Cyst fluid analysis:** epithelial cells rich in glycogen, very low levels of tumour markers.
- **Indications for resection:**
  - symptomatic;
  - biliary or pancreatic duct obstruction;
  - suspected malignancy;
  - increasing size on surveillance US/CT (every 6–12 months).

Mucinous cystic tumours

- 40–50% of cystic tumours.
- Cystadenoma and cystadenocarcinoma cannot be distinguished by pre-operative investigations and should therefore always be resected.
- 80% of mucinous cystadenomas are in the distal pancreas.
- Large cysts with septa.
- Peripheral calcification +/− solid intracystic component.
- Radiologically may appear similar to pseudocysts.
- A large unilocular cyst with no prior history of pancreatitis, in an otherwise normal pancreas is most likely to be a mucinous pancreatic neoplasm.
- If there is a history of pancreatitis (which can complicate mucinous tumours), examination of cyst fluid may discriminate between tumour and pseudocyst.
- **Cyst fluid analysis:** very low levels of pancreatic enzymes (amylase), high tumour markers, mucin-containing or malignant cells.
- **Misdiagnosis for pseudocyst:**
  - mucinous cystadenoma 9%;
  - mucinous cystadenocarcinoma 15%;
  - risk increases if the cystic tumour communicates through the pd;
  - treat by surgical resection.
- 5-year survival after resection of mucinous cystadenocarcinoma is 50%.

Intraductal papillary mucinous tumours
- 11% of cystic tumours.
- Duct lining produces a mucus secretion, which fills the lumen of pancreatic ducts, causing cystic dilatation of main or secondary branches.
- EUS or CT show duct dilatation with no obstructing lesion.
- Duodenoscopy shows mucus oozing from major papilla.
- Pancreatography shows numerous plugs in dilated pancreatic ducts.
- Histological analysis may show adenoma with dysplasia or adenocarcinoma.
- Treat by surgical resection.

Solid and papillary epithelial neoplasm
- 4% of cystic tumours.
- Also known as Frantz's tumour.
- Young women or adolescents. Median age of diagnosis is 27 years.
- Cystic areas consist of regions of haemorrhage and necrosis.
- Consider diagnosis in patient with a large tumour with solid and cystic areas, calcification and a capsule.
- MRI is superior to CT for diagnosis.
- Treat by surgical resection.
- 5-year survival after resection 97%.

Mucinous non-cystic or colloid Ca (1–3%)
Small published series.
- n = 17. >80% of tumour composed of colloic carcinoma (CC).
- Mean tumour diameter = 5.3cm.
- In >50%, CC represented the invasive component of a IPMT or mucinous cystic neoplasm.
- 57% 5 year survival.

Endocrine tumours

Classification

Endocrine microadenoma
Well differentiated pancreatic endocrine neoplasm
- **Functional:**
  - insulinoma;
  - glucagonoma;
  - somatostatinoma;
  - VIPoma (vasoactive intestinal peptide-secreting tumour);
  - gastrinoma;
  - carcinoid tumour;
  - other ectopic and mixed hormone producing neoplasms.
- **Non-functional:** PPoma (pancreatic polypeptide-secreting tumour).

Poorly differentiated endocrine carcinoma
- Small cell carcinoma.
- Large cell endocrine carcinoma.
- Mixed endocrine carcinoma.

Diagnosis and staging
- Functional hormone assays (see Neuroendocrine liver metastases, Pathology 📖 p. 160).
- Cross-sectional imaging (CT or MRI).
- **Tumour localization:**
  - somatostain receptor scintigraphy (also known as octreotide scan);
  - portal venous sampling.

Management
- Enucleate small encapsulated tumours <2cm.
- Resect if >2cm (distal pancreatectomy or Whipple's procedure).
- For management of liver metastases, see Neuroendocrine liver metastases 📖 p. 160).

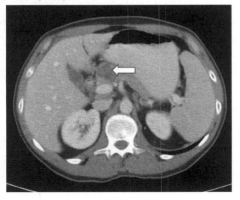

Fig. 11.4 Pancreatic neuroendocrine tumour.

Pancreatic trauma

- Rare, usually associated with significant deceleration injury or direct blow to epigastrium. Often associated with injury to left lobe of liver.
- Serum amylase is elevated in 85% of patients.
- Morbidity increased if main pancreatic duct injured or delayed diagnosis.

Grading of injury (Lucas system)

- **Grade I:** superficial contusion only.
- **Grade II:** deep laceration or transection of the left side of the pancreas.
- **Grade III:** injury to pancreatic head.

Initial management

- Diagnosis usually made by contrast-enhanced CT (free fluid, lesser sac collection, oedema, transection).
- Assess integrity of pancreatic duct (ERCP).
- If PD intact and patient stable → trial of non-operative management.
- If PD disrupted → surgery.

Surgical approach

- Enter lesser sac via gastrocolic omentum.
- Kocherize the duodenum.
- Retroperitoneal haematoma indicates possible pancreatic injury.
- **Grade I injury:** drainage only (pancreatic fistula rate 10–15%).
- **Grade II injury:** distal pancreatectomy or modified Puestow procedure.
- **Grade III injury:** repair associated major vascular injuries; damage control surgery in unstable, acidotic patients (e.g. drainage and planned re-look laparotomy at 48h).
- **Associated bile duct injury:** repair over T-tube or Roux-en-Y hepatico-jejunostomy.
- **Associated duodenal injury:** primary repair, duodenal exclusion, or Roux-en-Y as a closure.
- Pancreatico-duodenectomy is rarely indicated for pancreatic trauma.

Post-operative complications

- Pancreatic abscess.
- Pancreatic fistula.
- Pancreatic pseudocyst.

Pancreatico-duodenectomy (Whipple's procedure)

Incisions
- Rooftop.
- Upper transverse.
- Vertical midline.

Procedure
Determine resectability
- Kocherize duodenum to expose IVC. Confirm mobility of pancreatic tumour. Lift transverse colon to look for tumour infiltration at root of mesocolon.
- Enter lesser sac. Confirm the presence of a plane between SMV and neck of pancreas.

Dissection
- Perform cholecystectomy.
- Transect common hepatic duct above insertion of cystic duct (1cm distal to confluence of left and right hepatic ducts).
- Skeletonize the portal vein, preserving accessory right hepatic artery if present.
- Ligate and divide gastroduodenal artery.
- Resect all lymph nodes around common hepatic artery.
- Continue duodenal Kocherization to aortocaval recess and SMV.
- Ligate and divide the right gastroepiploic vessels.
- Resect distal third of stomach.
- Divide pancreatic neck.
- Mobilize duodenojejunal flexure and divide jejunum 15cm beyond it.
- Dissect uncinate processes off SMV and SMA, ligating all small branches and tributaries.

Reconstruction
- Create a 60cm Roux loop.
- Pancreatico-jejunostomy: duct-to-mucosa anastomosis using 5/0 or 6/0 PDS. Second layer of interrupted non-absorbable sutures between cut surface of pancreas and seromuscular layer of jejunal loop.
- Hepaticojejunostomy: end-to-side anastomosis using 5/0 PDS.
- Gastrojejunostomy: retrocolic side-to-side anastomosis.
- Jejuno-jejunosotomy: end-to-side anastomosis.
- Feeding jejunostomy.

Pylorus-preserving pancreaticoduodenectomy
- This modification of the classic Whipple procedure was introduced to reduce the incidence of post-operative dumping and bile reflux.
- Earlier studies suggested that PPPD is associated with an increased incidence of *delayed gastric emptying*.
- RCTs and meta-analyses have shown no difference in terms of cancer-related survival or post-operative mortality/morbidity between PPPD and Whipple's, although these studies are heterogeneous and underpowered.

Common pitfalls
Portal and/or superior mesenteric vein involved with tumour
- Resect portion of involved SMV or PV.
- If possible, close vein by primary repair (continuous 5/0 prolene).
- If the vein is too narrow, resect it, mobilize the proximal and distal ends, and perform end-to-end anastomosis (using autologous internal jugular vein graft if necessary).

Pancreatic resection margin involved with tumour
Mobilize pancreas off splenic vein and/or perform total pancreatectomy.

Post-operative care
- Adequate pain relief (epidural for 4 days).
- Early mobilization and DVT prophylaxis.
- Start enteral feeding via nasojejunal or feeding jejunostomy tube on day 1. Allow sips of water po.
- Increase oral fluids on day 3.
- Check amylase content in abdominal drains on day 4.
- Remove drains if no evidence of pancreatic, bile or chyle leak.

Post-operative complications
Pancreatic anastomotic leak
- Also called *pancreatic fistula*.
- Definition: drainage of >10mL/day of amylase-rich fluid on day 5 or for >5 days.
- Incidence 10–15%.
- Associated with increased morbidity/mortality and prolonged hospital stay.
- Varied clinical presentation:
  - opalescent fluid in surgical drain;
  - fever;
  - pain;
  - ileus;
  - gastric outlet obstruction;
  - sepsis;
  - secondary haemorrhage from ruptured pseudoaneurysm.
- Diagnosis: send drain fluid for biochemical analysis of amylase content (elevated in; US/CT-guided drainage of new intra-abdominal collections.

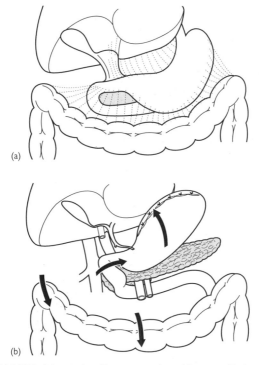

Fig. 11.5 Whipple's procedure. Key steps are indicated. Dissection. Kocherization of the duodenum; cholecystectomy; division of the gastrocolic omentum; mobilization and division of the duodenojejunal flexure; division of the distal stomach; division of the neck of the pancreas; mobilization of the head of the pancreas off portal vein/superior mesenteric vein and artery. Reconstruction. Retrocolic Roux-en-Y hepatico-jejunostomy (single-layer interrupted 5/0 PDS), pancreatico-jejunostomy in two layers: duct-to-mucosa (6/0 PDS) and serosa-to-capsule (4/0 PDS). Jejunos-jejunostomy (two layers 3/0 PDS; gastrojejunostomy (two layers 3/0 PDS).

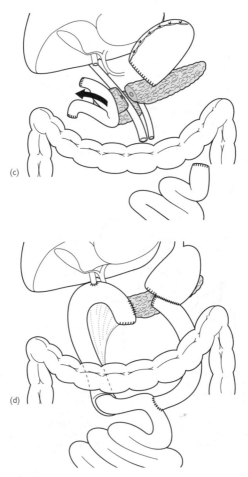

Fig. 11.5 (Contd).

- Minor pancreatic fistula (grade A) with no clinical sequelae with no radiological evidence of collections do not require any specific treatment.
- Pancreatic fistula associated with persistent (>3 weeks) leak (grade B) should be treated by NBM, parenteral feeding +/− SC octreotide.
- Pancreatic fistula associated with systemic signs of sepsis (grade C) require aggressive treatment: HDU/ITU support, NBM, parenteral feeding, SC octreotide, antibiotics, drainage of collections.

- Grade C pancreatic fistulae are associated with prolonged hospital stay, septic complications and mortality. Rarely, surgical intervention may be required if the patient deteriorates despite maximal conservative therapy. Surgical options include:
  - conversion from pancreatico-jejunostomy to pancreaticogastrostomy;
  - debridement and drainage;
  - completion pancreatectomy.

Delayed gastric emptying
- Need to exclude mechanical obstruction and pancreatic fistula as underlying causes.
- Presents with large nasogastric aspirates, vomiting or distension.
- Confirm diagnosis, and exclude obstruction or pancreatic fistula by arranging CT with oral contrast and/or water-soluble contrast meal.
- Most cases resolve with conservative management: IV metoclopramide, IV erythromycin, nasogastric drainage, parenteral, or nasojejunal feeding.
- Treat associated pancreatic fistula (see previous).
- Treat obstruction by radiological or endoscopic balloon dilatation of the gastrojejunal anastomosis.
- Rarely, a technical error may require revisional surgery.

Haemorrhage
- Significant bleeding associated with shock in the first 24h indicates technical error (e.g. slipped ligature) and should be treated by immediate reoperation.
- Secondary haemorrhage (intra-abdominal or gastrointestinal) after 5–10 days is often due to a ruptured pseudoaneurysm in relation to a pancreatic leak and/or sepsis. Other causes include bleeding from the gastrojejunal anastomosis or peptic ulcer. Arrange urgent CT angiography and/or endoscopy. Treat by urgent angiography and selective embolization (see Fig. 2.6). Arrange urgent laparotomy if:
  - patient too unstable for angiography;
  - embolization unsuccessful;
  - angiography facilities are not available.

Chyle leak
- The volume of leak depends on the extent of lymphadenectomy and calibre of lymphatic channels that are disrupted.
- Ensure adequate drainage.
- Treat by low fat diet or medium chain fatty acids.

Bile leak
- Potential sources of bile leak:
  - bilio-enteric anastomosis;
  - jejunojejunal anastomosis.
- Exclude disconnection/necrosis of bilio-enteric anastomosis (lack of bile pigment in stool).
- Ensure adequate drainage.
- Antibiotics +/– antifungal therapy.
- Vast majority resolve with conservative management.
- For persistent, high volume leaks, consider percutaneous transhepatic biliary drainage +/– stenting across the bilio-enteric anastomosis, or surgical exploration.

Distal pancreatectomy

Incision
- Transverse.
- Bilateral subcostal.
- Laparoscopic.

Procedure
- Exclude peritoneal and/or liver metastases.
- Enter lesser sac via incision in gastrocolic omentum.
- Assess resectability of tumour.
- Incise peritoneum at inferior border of body of pancreas.
- Mobilize distal pancreas from underlying structures.
- Identify, doubly ligate, and divide the splenic vein on the posterior aspect of the pancreas at the point of transection.
- Identify, doubly ligate and divide the splenic artery on the superior border of the pancreas.
- Pass a nylon tape between the pancreas and the portal/superior mesenteric veins. Divide the pancreas with point diathermy.
- Identify and suture ligate the proximal end of the divided pancreatic duct using 5/0 PDS.
- Continue mobilizing the distal pancreas towards the spleen.
- Mobilize the spleen by ligating and dividing the short gastric vessels, and divide the lienorenal ligament.
- Achieve haemostasis.
- Place a medium-sized tube drain (24 or 28F) in the pancreatic bed.

Postoperative care
- Adequate pain relief (epidural for 4 days).
- 3 doses of prophylactic antibiotics. Convert to oral penicillin (lifelong post-splenectomy).
- Early mobilization and DVT prophylaxis.
- Start oral fluids on day 1. Return to normal diet as tolerated.
- Check amylase content in abdominal drain on day 4.
- Remove drain if no evidence of pancreatic or chyle leak.
- Immunize against *Pneumococcus*, *Haemophilus influenza* B and *Meningococcus* prior to discharge if not given preoperatively.
- Give patient post-splenectomy advice card and bracelet.
- Advise patient to have annual influenza vaccine.

Post-operative complications
- Bleeding.
- Wound infection.
- Intra-abdominal abscess.
- Pancreatic fistula.
- Post-splenectomy complications (e.g. infection).

Laparoscopic distal pancreatectomy

- Indications: benign tumours or cysts in distal pancreas.
- Avoids morbidity associated with a long upper abdominal scar; shorter hospital stay (no RCTs have been performed to compare with open technique).
- **Patient position:** supine, legs in lithotomy position, table tilted at 20° left side up.
- **Ports:** umbilical port for camera; 4 other ports in upper abdomen.
- **Dissection:** as per open technique. Divide pancreas with vascular stapler.

Spleen-preserving distal pancreatectomy

- Avoids potential post-splenectomy complications.
- Technically more demanding than standard distal pancreatectomy.
- **Indications:** benign tumours or cysts in distal pancreas.
- **Contraindications:** invasive cancer.
- Mobilize the pancreas from the splenic artery and vein; ligate and divide small branches.
- Dissect pancreatic tail from splenic hilum, taking care to avoid injuring splenic vessels.
- Divide pancreas as per standard distal pancreatectomy.

Longitudinal pancreatico-jejunostomy

Incision
Transverse or bilateral subcostal.

Procedure
- Puestow procedure (Fig. 11.6) or Partington-Rochelle (Fig. 11.7) modification.
- Enter lesser sac by incising gastrocolic omentum.
- Locate main pancreatic duct by palpation or aspirating with a 21G needle directed towards the pancreatic tail to avoid puncture of the portal vein.
- Incise the capsule of the pancreas overlying the pancreatic duct using point diathermy.
- Deepen the incision through pancreatic tissue and open the duct longitudinally. Debris and calculi are removed from the pancreatic duct.
- According to the original description by *Puestow*, the tail of the pancreas should be amputated, splenectomy performed, and the body and tail of the pancreas invaginated into a Roux limb of jejunum. These steps are omitted in the modified Puestow procedure (*Partington-Rochelle* modification), which describes a long side-to-side anastomosis between the filleted pancreatic duct and the Roux limb of jejunum (either duct-mucosa or capsule-mucosa).

Post-operative complications
- Bleeding.
- Pancreatic fistula.
- Infection.
- Recurrent or persistent pain.

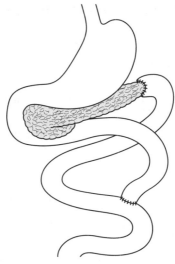

Fig. 11.6 Puestow procedure. Splenectomy and distal pancreatectomy. Tail of pancreas invaginated into and anastomosed to Roux-en-Y loop of jejunum.

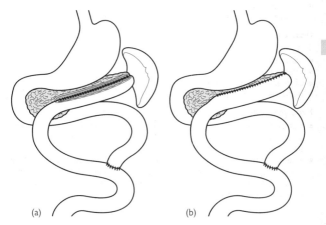

(a)

(b)

Fig. 11.7 Partington-Rochelle modification. Pancreatic duct is identified and opened longitudinally. Stones and debris are removed. Longitudinal pancreatico-jejunostomy.

Beger procedure (duodenum-preserving pancreatic head resection)

Incision
Transverse or bilateral subcostal.

Procedure
- Expose pancreatic head by incising the gastrocolic omentum.
- Divide the duodenocolic ligament.
- Kocherize the duodenum.
- Expose the superior mesenteric vein at the inferior border of the pancreas.
- Ligate and divide the gastroduodenal artery.
- Isolate and sling the common bile duct at the superior border of the duodenum.
- Pass a nylon tape behind the pancreatic neck.
- Divide the pancreatic neck to the right of the portal vein/superior mesenteric vein using point diathermy.
- Mobilize the pancreatic head from the portal vein, common bile duct and duodenum, carefully ligating small portal vein branches, and avoiding injury to these structures.
- Construct a retrocolic Roux loop and anastomose the jejunum to the residual pancreas, in two layers (duct-mucosa and capsule-serosa).
- Anastomose the residual pancreatic head to the Roux loop via a separate enterotomy
- If the distal common bile duct is strictured, a side-to-side choledochojejunostomy should also be performed.

Post-operative complications
- Bleeding.
- Pancreatic fistula.
- Infection.
- Bilio-enteric anastomotic stricture.
- Recurrent or persistent pain.

Frey procedure
- Failure to adequately decompress an obstructed proximal pancreatic duct is a common reason for persistent pain after *longitudinal pancreatico-jejunostomy*.
- The Frey procedure aims to decompress the entire pancreatic duct by combining a duodenum-preserving pancreatic head resection (Beger procedure) with a longitudinal pancreatico-jejunostomy (Partington-Rochelle modification of the Puestow procedure).

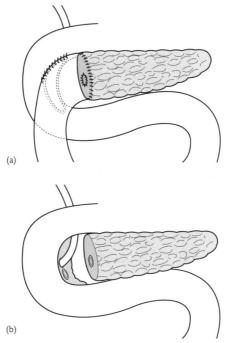

(a)

(b)

Fig. 11.8 Head of pancreas is removed, preserving common bile duct and rim of tissue adjacent to duodenum. Roux-en-Y jejunal loop fashioned and anastomosed to body of pancreas in two layers (as for Whipple's procedure) and to remnant pancreatic head.

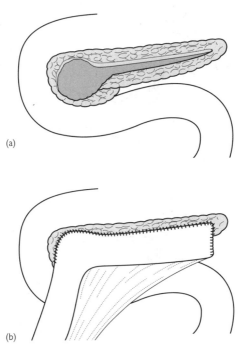

Fig. 11.9 Frey procedure Pancreatic duct is opened along its full length. Head of pancreas is cored out (as for Beger procedure). Longitudinal pancreatico-jejunostomy.

Index